TUNA BREATH

Dear Barbara,

Thank you for entering the Goodreads Book Giveaway for "Tuna Breath" — and congrats on winning this copy!

Enjoy :)

Doug Poulsen
08/13

TUNA BREATH

A 275-POUND TEENAGER'S COMING OF AGE STORY

DOUG PEDERSEN

BALBOA.
PRESS

A DIVISION OF HAY HOUSE

Balboa Press books may be ordered through booksellers or by contacting:

Balboa Press
A Division of Hay House
1663 Liberty Drive
Bloomington, IN 47403
www.balboapress.com
1-(877) 407-4847

Because of the dynamic nature of the Internet, any web addresses or links contained in this book may have changed since publication and may no longer be valid. The views expressed in this work are solely those of the author and do not necessarily reflect the views of the publisher, and the publisher hereby disclaims any responsibility for them.

The author of this book does not dispense medical advice or prescribe the use of any technique as a form of treatment for physical, emotional, or medical problems without the advice of a physician, either directly or indirectly. The intent of the author is only to offer information of a general nature to help you in your quest for emotional and spiritual well-being. In the event you use any of the information in this book for yourself, which is your constitutional right, the author and the publisher assume no responsibility for your actions.

Any people depicted in stock imagery provided by Thinkstock are models, and such images are being used for illustrative purposes only. Certain stock imagery © Thinkstock.

Printed in the United States of America.

ISBN: 978-1-4525-7579-7 (sc)
ISBN: 978-1-4525-7580-3 (e)

Balboa Press rev. date: 07/10/2013

For my entire family—without every one of you, my healing
would not have been possible, nor would *Tuna Breath*.

And special thanks to my mother for always knowing,
nurturing, encouraging, and loving me . . . no matter what.

CONTENTS

INTRODUCTION

Obesity is defined as having an excessive amount of body fat. Doctors often use a formula based on your height and weight—called the body mass index (BMI)—to determine if you are obese. [People] with a BMI of 30 or higher are considered obese.

—Mayo Clinic Staff

Being fat is an *individual* emotional problem. Being a fat teenager is a *shared* emotional problem that includes the parents—especially *Mom*. That's why I wrote this book.

From my perspective, the emotional aspects of being a fat teenager (of being obese) are hardly emphasized at all. Turn on the TV, read websites, or check out the latest books and you'll see trainers, teachers, counselors, doctors, and weight loss success stories all talking about calories, food choices, and exercise. Don't get me wrong; those things are vitally important. However, I know firsthand that the key, the real success to helping a teenager (a child) with a serious weight problem, requires much more than just a food and exercise plan.

My experience as a super-fat kid started way before "obesity" was a common description for seriously overweight people. I was seven years old. It was the 1980s and before grunge music, the Internet, or renewable anything. Gastric bypasses weren't performed and drug makers weren't advertising on TV. *The Real World* was the only reality TV show, and we didn't yet know about *The Biggest Loser*. There weren't any obese kids either. There were only small handfuls of *super fat kids* like me at each school.

I consistently gained massive amounts of weight for about ten years. Topping out at 275 pounds in high school was the largest accomplishment

I thought I'd ever have. All my dreams were dead. I seriously thought that I would be 500 pounds someday. I didn't know that my obesity was meeting my own human needs for certainty and significance in life. I didn't know that inadequacy, self-pity, and self-loathing were forms of significance that allowed me to connect to myself—albeit in the most negative ways. I didn't know that my keys to freedom rested in meeting my human needs for love, growth, and contribution. As a result, I was deeply insecure throughout those *super fat* years, which led me to feel alone and privately unhappy most of the time.

Fortunately, my environment changed when I was eighteen years old. This was the first of three major turning points I describe in the book. I didn't have a coach or doctors to help, so I starved myself and lost 125 pounds in eight months. Along the way, I learned about my own body, desire, sacrifice, and self-discipline. *Turning Point #1* was all about seeking *physical balance*.

You can imagine how happy I must have been. Ironically, from that point forward, I acted very confident (even arrogant) and pursued my life's ambitions. I joined the US Marine Corps and became a hard-charging war machine. I binged on this lifestyle. Deep on the inside, however, I was still running from my past. I hid things about myself, I was rigid with people, and I was still that sensitive, sometimes insecure, and privately unhappy soul most of the time. By the time I left the Marines, my emotions were still *way out of whack*. I was aggressive, quick to show anger, and hated certain people for little or no good reason.

Turning Point #2 occurred when I finally acknowledged that my unhappiness (my hate) was my fault and when I decided to try to find a way to change my reactions/attitudes towards people. *TP #2* was all about seeking *emotional balance*. Seeking emotional balance isn't an easy task; at least not for me at the ripe old age of twenty-four.

After the Marines, I graduated college and pursued Wall Street and investment banking before eventually finding some success as a corporate salesperson. Since being super fat, I had achieved everything I had ever set my mind to, yet I was still lonely, empty, and deeply unhappy. I didn't know at first that the same emotional drivers that had contributed to my obesity had followed me into my young adult and adult life. There's no doubt they were fully present and powerful. However, instead of using food to binge and meet my needs, over time I substituted aggression, alcohol, relationships with random girls, and the pursuit of money, bingeing on those things instead.

Turning Point #3 occurred when I acknowledged this reality. My veil of blindness finally started to lift when I saw my life (my struggle) as it really was: my creation. *TP #3* was all about healing the past . . . about seeking *wholeness*.

Since then, I've learned that my well-developed binge-eating habits and personality were a *low-road* way for me to meet my own human needs; it was how I negatively connected to myself for a long time. This is a key reason for deciding to tell my story, for I believe this is the risk for seriously overweight teens (and their parents) if they don't get their emotional houses in order. Specifically, several things are likely to occur if mothers don't help their teens or if the children can't tackle their emotional drivers on their own:

- They never improve their health and actually get worse (physically and emotionally).
- They lose weight but regress (yo-yo dieting).
- They lose weight permanently but continue to project other binge-eating types of behaviors as they mature (as I did).

Please keep in mind that *Tuna Breath* is not a "how-to" book. Someday soon, I will write a specific how-to book that details the four phases/actions in my coaching program. But for now, Mom should expect to *go deep* if she wants to successfully help her teenager with his weight problem—with his life. Because success really lies with loosening the *death grip* that inadequacy and self-pity has on her child. Simply put, Mom must prepare to help the child do the following:

- Understand their basic human needs structure
- Identify their specific triggers and patterns
- Analyze and rewrite their *rules*
- Neutralize their destructive vice(s)

Tuna Breath is a "how I" story. It's my starting point and a "can do!" message for you, my reader. It shines a light on the bigger, deeper issue of weight loss and exposes the long-term emotional risks that overweight children face. My specific story should be a metaphor for some to learn from. You can always count on my sincere honesty and my all-access approach to telling the real story. My writing is sometimes funny, sarcastic, ironic, heated, or repetitive. I do this for a purpose. I want it to strike an emotional chord, so I also use language and word choices that are slang or that may seem aggressive at times.

My true intention is to inspire moms and their seriously overweight children to improve their personal foundations. Hopefully, my readers are moved to self-analyze in a new way—in a new light. And ultimately, I want moms to understand and fully connect to their children, to communicate differently, to learn from my mistakes, and to help their children save the time that I wasted.

Thank you for reading my story!

Doug P.

CHAPTER 1

LIKE "NURSE" WITH AN "-ISS"

The only certainties in life are "time" and "change." The question you must ask yourself: is now the time to change?

—Doug Pedersen

D o you remember your last first date? I certainly remember mine. My last first date was with a woman named Nurys Maria. She was Dominican and spoke with a half-Spanish and half-Brooklyn accent—an attractive Virgo with a quick wit. I thought it was cute when she would say "boss" or "balls." Like many New Yorkers, she would drawl certain words out with an *au* sound, such as when you say the word "Au-gust." Boss turned into *bauss*, and balls turned into *baulls.* "My *bauss* has *baulls* as big as church bells! Adios mio, mi amor!" she would never say.

Most people either really love or really hate dating. There's hardly any middle ground, which I always found fascinating. The people who love dating are the ones who eventually escape the game by getting married—at least the married people I know. The ones who hate dating are the *forever singles.* How can there be so many single people on earth who can't seem to find each other? They all seemingly want the same thing. They're right next to each other. They can physically see each other. They can even talk to each other. But they just can't seem to *find* each other. Fascinating!

1

One buddy used to tell me that dating was like a game: You win some and you lose some. There's always the thrill of the hunt. You can score points or get thrown in the penalty box. Another used to describe it like fishing: reel one in, watch it squirm a bit, and either keep it in the boat or toss it back into the ocean. I always thought dating was like work . . . or maybe I thought work was like dating. Either way, I always felt that going on a date was like going on a job interview, which I proved to be pretty good at. In some instances, I felt that dating was like being interrogated in a prison camp, which I had also been trained for and was apparently pretty good at.

Like anybody before a first date, I had the typical anxieties with Nurys Maria. I wondered how well we would get along. Was she going to like the lunch spot I picked? Would she think I was funny? What if we didn't have anything in common? How honest should I be with her? How vulnerable should I be, if at all? What was my bailout plan if the date was a bust? Should I try to kiss her if it went well? It didn't help that I practically had to beg her to go out with me. So much work for a simple lunch date. I just wanted to have lunch with her and see if we were second date (night date) worthy. "So tell me again, *Daug*. Just what *exactly* do you want to do again? Just what *exactly* are your intentions again?" she said repeatedly during the phone conversation that took ninety playful but frustrating minutes.

Nurys Maria's accent was definitely not her most unique feature. As it turned out, she immigrated to America in the late eighties, as my grandpa had done from Denmark in the thirties. She was naturally intelligent and was blessed with a good set of street smarts too. She told me how she decided to go to college in New York City. She stayed after that, and over time, she became a citizen and a successful professional. She had long legs and a figure like a well-crafted Spanish guitar. Her olive skin was creamy, and I could tell that she took care of herself because her arms and shoulders were also toned. I liked her smile, when I could get her to crack one, and I could see myself getting lost at some point in her long curly black hair. Her big brown eyes were genuine and sharp, like an eagle's; she didn't miss anything. Her full Virgo lips were quick to shoot a dart or command an answer to any compromising direct question. "So tell me again, really, have you killed anyone or what?" she asked during some "light" conversation as we sat in a chocolate bar sipping cocoa on our first date on Michigan Avenue.

Nurys Maria was different from anyone I had dated before. She was a real woman, an adult, and not the typical pasty girl that I had gone for in the past. Not that I wasn't pasty. With my blond hair and blue eyes, I looked like Casper the featureless ghost in many pictures. Thankfully, I had a chance to test, and tell, her about her womanhood one day before our date. My little experiment gave me the impression that she wasn't the type to fall for cheesy pickup lines that were dreamed up in the twisted bowels of a dark Irish pub. Hers was a natural beauty that many guys would notice and act on. Charm would only take me so far. If I was going to get anywhere with her, I was going to have to be as unique and as smart as she was.

They also say that you never get a second chance to make a good first impression. Having had a flash encounter several months before our date, thankfully I had two chances with Nurys Maria to make an impression. The first was at a fund-raiser downtown. I was with a good female friend of mine from college, and we acted as if we were the next hot comedy team to hit Vegas. It didn't bother me if we looked a little obnoxious; we had many laughs, inside jokes, and classy high (and yes, low) fives. Our joke of the night was her cell phone, which she had carried to the party in a clear plastic baggie full of white rice. She had taken a seemingly important call from the shower a few days prior, which *shockingly* damaged her phone. Friends of ours had counseled her that it could be fixed using the white rice trick. Apparently, the rice would absorb the moisture like a sponge and she'd be back in business. None of us thought she would carry it to the party, though, especially not me . . . And I thought I was the blond.

My friend and I stopped at the first table in the room because it was closest to the vodka line; I always made sure of that. There were several other people at the round cocktail table, and we each took turns introducing ourselves. I noticed Nurys Maria immediately. She was so different from the Midwest girls at the party that I couldn't help but stare. She was standing there with a Latino guy who introduced himself as Oscar, and then it was her turn. She said, "Nurys—like 'nurse' with an '-iss.'"

Oscar rudely interrupted my gaze and asked me what I did for a living. With a big sarcastic smile, I looked directly at Nurys Maria and with a wink said, "I sell computer hardware, software, and services to enterprise customers. How about you, pretty lady?"

"I just *baught* an HP printer," she darted back as her eyes rolled to the left and away from me. After a few more boring pleasantries, I carried on with the party. My friend and I continued to make as much of a scene as possible while spending more time in the vodka line. Several hours later, while trolling by the chocolate fondue station, I noticed that my good buddy Oscar had left the lovely Nurys Maria unattended. I was puzzled. *How could you leave a woman like that by herself at a gala?* I thought. *Rookie move!* She did not look happy. In fact, she looked crampy. *Whatever it is they have, it can't be anything serious,* I thought. So I made my move.

I approached her bearing tiny sweet gifts. Still, the tension was so thick that I needed more than strawberries; I could've used a chainsaw. She stared me down like a state trooper running radar as I walked smartly across the ballroom. I must have looked like a Doberman in heat because I could feel her inner Virgo ready to fillet me like a red snapper as I got closer. She was probably used to beating back the lame flirty gestures guys often threw at her, but I just couldn't resist. Something deep in my primal being told me that I needed to compete for this woman.

I moved my body close to hers and spoke softly in her ear. "Hey there, you! I couldn't help but notice that you're standing here all alone."

"Yeah?" she fired back as both of her eyes threatened another death roll.

"Well, I just wanted to come over here and let you know that I think you are the most beautiful woman in this room." She didn't move away, so I stepped in a little closer "And I mean, by far the most beautiful I've seen. You're all woman, man! Chocolate strawberry?"

This was not my best work, not that I was intending to melt her heart or anything. I just wanted to express myself to her. I knew that I could be a little obnoxious at times, and even arrogant, but the fun part for me was that I meant every word of it. I didn't lie to girls; I didn't have to. Nurys Maria was a woman in a room full of girls—a real woman—and I could see it. So what if Oscar saw her first? I thought dating was like a sport, and there's nothing wrong with a little healthy competition, right?

My irresistible charm did not get me a date with Nurys Maria that night. After I laid my egg, we parted ways. I didn't get her number. I didn't know what she did. I didn't know where she came from. I didn't know where she lived. And although someone had told me, I couldn't remember which one of her friends at the party was also my friend. She was the mystery woman. I quickly moved on, but it was hard to forget Nurys—like "nurse" with an "-iss."

My redemption came a few months later. I was sitting in the bar sipping my usual vodka soda at a popular Chicago restaurant, waiting for the group to show up. I wasn't really excited about the night's events because I was waiting for my "C group"—the group I hung out with when my "A group" and "B group" were tied up. They were good people, though, and I felt bad at times for labeling them Cs. But labeling groups seemed so natural to me after learning to do this with my customer account list, even though I was trying to break that habit with people. I had met most of the Cs through volunteering at the food bank or at the homeless shelter. They all seemed to live much calmer lives than I did. I was more of a swashbuckler in my free time and enjoyed getting rowdy in the wee hours. I never told them this, but my time spent volunteering was usually an effort to make amends for my digressions of times past.

The Cs filtered in one at a time, and I greeted them each with my customary hug. I'm a big hugger, and after I gave my last one, I saw her in the short distance. Nurys Maria walked through the rotating door, and I felt my face light up like the New Year's Eve sky. "Heeyyy, you! You're that girl from the party!" I said with a wink as I went in for the hug.

"You mean *woman*, don't you, Don Juan?" she cracked back with her warm Caribbean smile and her big brown eyes wide open.

What a twist of events, I thought. The night is definitely looking up! Someone had invited her, and I just knew that I needed to compete—again. Of all the Cs, she was bound to be my best conversation at the table, so I had to make sure that I sat next to her at dinner.

After a few more pleasantries and a couple of one-liners, we started to walk back to the round table for ten that waited for us. I asked her to save me a seat while I hit the men's, and as if we'd known each other for ten years, she fired back, "What, do you have a small bladder or something?"

Oh, it was on after that! The games had begun. My smile beamed like the sun as I walked to the bathroom, stood at the urinal, and talked myself up in the mirror before heading back to the Cs. *Smart, beautiful, and witty,* too, I thought.

I was happy to see that she'd saved me a seat, and I made sure to talk in her ear the whole night. Actually, I listened the whole night. My talking consisted mainly of asking many open-ended questions, another technique that I learned in sales. Plus, learning about her was fun—like gathering intelligence before a sniper mission. I listened to her answers about New York, about being new to Chicago, about her love of the Gipsy Kings' music, and about starting a business. I got to know her, and I didn't let up until she relinquished her business card. I gave her mine as well, and I learned later that she immediately threw it away that night. I also learned that she didn't even know Oscar at all. He was just some *chooch* that happened to be at the same party as us months before. Nurys Maria actually thought he was with me and believed it was a setup when Oscar asked, "So, what do you do?"

With much persistence on my part, we had many dates after that. One of my favorite dates was a brunch trip to China Town on a lazy Saturday in 2007. Although she was Dominican, she raved about the fact that it was the year of the Pig. "Woo-hoo, it's my year! It's my year!" she would sing out of nowhere. I didn't know about astrology or the zodiac at all, although I knew that I was an Aquarius. I also didn't follow the Chinese calendar before meeting Nurys Maria, although I learned later that I was a Tiger. With all the excitement about her year, I thought it would be fun to sip Heinekens and eat dim sum with the locals. Thankfully, she agreed, and although I was trusted with a Top Secret clearance in the Marine Corps, I willfully told every "ancient Chinese secret" that I knew while we drove to brunch. *Ancient Chinaman say, "Man with hand in pocket feel cocky all day!"*

Neither of us had been to Chicago's Chinatown before. When we got there, we walked through a courtyard that had twelve stone statues, each representing an animal for every month in the Chinese calendar. Since she was a Pig, I asked her if she wanted me to take a picture of her next to the Pig statue with my cell phone. She thought that was an excellent idea and quickly struck her best model pose: cheeks sunken in, lips pouted, chin down and chest up, hands on her hips, slim tummy, torso slightly twisted, and her legs crossed. I took my hands out of my pocket and readied the camera.

"Hey, wait a minute. Are you sure you're a Pig?" I knew I sounded puzzled as I pulled the phone down and squinted at the statue. Like a bad "Heard on the Street" quote, this wasn't a great question to ask a beautiful woman out in the open while on a date, but the statue listed all the years of the Pig. She had told me weeks before that that she was born in 1973. The statue said that Pigs were born in 1971, the same year as my older brother by two years. Oops!

After that, I knew that Nurys Maria and I, at the very least, would be friends forever. I had caught her in a little white lie—and it was about her age, no less. I never would have asked a classy woman about her age in the first place. Still, I couldn't help but tease her about it. Had the situation been reversed, she would never have let me live it down. But she was vulnerable to me now—at least a little bit—and I wondered what else we would learn about each other that would feel uncomfortable, build trust, pull us apart, or keep us together.

I felt uncomfortable about plenty of things—even insecure about some. I carried a brash persona in front of her, and in general, but I wondered if she would stop going out with me if she saw my pale white dimpled butt up close. I was in shape, but what if it made her laugh or even gag? I had managed to get this far in life with it, but I was also self-conscious about it. What would I do then? At one point, we started signing our e-mails with funny names that only we thought were cute. Mine was *Superhombre*. What would she do if she saw the eighteen-inch scar that stretched across my abdomen—the best reminder of my tummy tuck? What would she do if she learned how I really got it? What would she do if she saw my jealousy? What would she do once she saw every side of me?

Being vulnerable wasn't something I really ever strived for. I had tried letting my insecurities show in front of a girl once before, and I didn't like how I slept after that. Plus, my older brother had a few heart-wrenching breakups when we were younger. These were the kinds of breakups that made you want to take twenty shots of tequila on dollar night at the local alehouse. His breakups were, like, *Old Yeller* sad. They were bad, and I told myself that I never wanted any part of that agony.

I rarely showed my vulnerabilities after that. I had an answer for everything and considered myself a smooth operator. Like most guys I know, I had spent a lot of years building up different experiences and attitudes that didn't really lend to being sensitive and caring when it came to certain things. But the truth of the matter was that at my core, behind my male ego, rested a deep sea of sensitivities to things that I cared passionately about—and felt vulnerable about. Hardly anybody knew these deep secrets about me because I hid them very well. Who could ever accept me for them, let alone love me for them? I often wondered. Only my close family members and some old friends knew the whole me—and even that was questionable at times.

I didn't become vulnerable to Nurys Maria until six or seven months after our first date. It was more spontaneous actually, but I had been working on my issues for a while, and I thought that I would take a chance. I always liked a good risk, but I still felt a little scared as I considered letting her in on all of who I was. *What if she judges me for it and I lose her?* I wondered. I didn't have the confidence in myself or in my story before that to place my bets and let the chips fall where they may when it came to love. You know, tell her the truth and feel okay with any reaction she had. Instead of feeling secure in who I was, I wanted to hold on and keep her image of me the way I wanted her to see it, just as I had done with lots of people over my life. It was like being a Broadway actor—Anthony Hopkins or Edward Norton, perhaps. Or maybe I was more like Eddie Haskell.

I remember that when I told her, we were boyfriend and girlfriend already. I had asked her to be mine on a similar morning that summer. "*Whut du yu tink a-but bng my girh-freinh?*" I muddled out as I casually brushed my teeth. It was pathetic because my mouth was full of toothpaste and my lips were covered in white foam like a rabid dog or a Doberman in heat. I could never keep my toothpaste where it belonged: on my teeth and in my mouth. Or maybe I brushed harder as the nervous anxiety in my stomach swirled while I waited for her to answer.

I was a little surprised when she actually said yes. We had been exclusive since we met, but we had never really talked about our relationship. What relationship? She resisted me so much at first. She didn't even want to date at all—nobody. And me, I was more like a teenage boy who couldn't commit to anything or anybody. We were both so cynical about the opposite sex when we first met that we never even used the R-word.

What we did talk about that morning was my discipline. Nurys Maria knew that I liked to exercise, and she had spent enough time around me to know that I paid attention to the foods that I ate, although she also wondered why I didn't do the same with the vodka sodas I often drank. She made a few comments about how consistent I was—how good I was with my food and how I never cheated—and she wondered how I could work so hard and still drag myself to the gym to get my workouts in week after week.

In that moment, I decided to do something that I had never done before with a woman. I felt that this story was coming, but I had been reluctant to tell it in fear that she might judge me (as I had felt about telling anybody who didn't know me really, really well.) But I wanted to be honest with my new girlfriend, so I decided to place my bets and let the chips fall where they may.

In a low voice I said, "Well, I was really fat as a kid, and I lost a ton of weight after high school."

The butterflies swirled in my stomach the instant "I was really fat" left my lips. What had I just blurted out? *Why did I just do that?* I wondered. I had kept this kind of information locked away in my "safe," only to be shared with people who knew me for much longer periods of time. In fact, I hadn't shared it with some people who had known me for ten years. Why would I? I always thought that skinny people judged fat people. They made fun of us behind our backs and even to our faces. We looked funny, had odd odors, perspired at the wrong times, and couldn't hide our shame.

When I was fat, they didn't call us obese. Obesity wasn't talked about very often and not ever in public. Fat people were just fat. They were people who were lazy, with no self-control; they couldn't control their appetites; they had a hanker'n for Grandma's cook'n. Fat people never had cool clothes that fit well or dated the cute girls, if they dated at all. Fat people had emotional issues. And if you were a really fat kid, these judgments, these insecurities, would multiply through your heart and soul like a global epidemic.

I knew that she could feel the gravity of my honesty, for she gently probed a little more. "Really? How did you do it, sweetie?" she asked.

At first, I tried to make it sound as if it were because I played football. But wanting to build even more trust with her, I quickly caved to my uncomfortable place of vulnerability. I told her how I had dropped my weight in a short time by eating (more like starving) as if I were on a deserted island, limiting my diet to tuna and oranges every day. She looked puzzled and curious, so I didn't stop there. My fear rippled my skin as I went on to tell her that I had gained my weight because of an ugly period in my childhood. I told her how my dad was sent to the hospital; how our family was rejected by our church like a turd stew before hitting hard times; and how I lived in fear that our perfect family was going to shatter like a mirror.

I gave her details about that dreadful time that I had never talked about with anyone outside my family—ever. I hadn't talked about it in decades. This conversation happened so fast. It was scary because I didn't know how she was going to react. I knew that I didn't want her to see the sensitive fat kid when she looked at me . . . or wonder who I really was. But I had just exposed a deep piece of my soul to her, and I crossed my fingers as I wondered what she would think, and do, next.

CHAPTER 2

DON'T BE AN OXYMORON

Hope is the fuel that raises our standards. Losing it deletes our most basic desires.

—Doug Pedersen

I don't know about you, but I've never felt that I was the smartest person in the room. Not that I've ever felt dumb; it's just that since I was a kid in grammar school, no one's ever accused me of being the brightest bulb on the tree, the sharpest knife in the drawer, or the one you want to copy off of in class—if you know what I mean. I suppose you could say that I was a bit of a slacker when it came to academics.

I was selective, I suppose, and only focused on things I felt interested in. Like picking a good restaurant or swinging at a good pitch. You don't pick a place that serves nasty food, and you don't swing your bat at a wild pitch. So why concentrate on things that you don't like—like homework? That's how my young brain worked in the 1980s and early '90s.

Most of the time I thought sitting in a classroom was like watching a soap opera: nothing said was relevant to my life, and the conversations were as interesting as yarn. In any given class in any given grade, you could assume that I was daydreaming about anything but schoolwork, cracking jokes, talking in the back of the class, or ditching school altogether. While other kids recited their times tables, I often looked around the room and thought about which kid I was going to peg in dodgeball during recess. While teachers passed out assignments, I would often daydream about how cool it would be to go swimming at my friend's house, especially if I could fly there on a magic carpet first. If I missed an assignment, no problem! I had no shame in asking a fellow kid for a hand up. "Hey, guy, you know what would be cool? If you let me copy your homework!"

By the time I was in high school, I learned how to forge absentee notes and get out of class without being a truant. I remember one time driving to school when I was sixteen years old. I had just gotten my license and was proud while rollin' down the street in my '72 Oldsmobile Cutlass. It was made of steel, and I felt it was a real chick magnet. Actually, it only attracted crumbs from the food I spilled in it, but it was mine, and it gave me freedom. The bench seat was especially nice because my luscious love handles and bodacious buttocks could spread comfortably across it. I also had installed six-by-nine-inch speakers that I could crank Guns N' Roses tapes (yes, tapes—I had a tape case too) when not listening to morning radio on the way to school.

The radio show that I listened to broke for a commercial. I immediately started to scan for other music, and a man's voice filled the airwaves. He had a New York accent, and his voice was deep and sharp—like James Earl Jones's. Then he unexpectedly shocked me when he said, "I'll give you fifty bucks to show me your vagina right now! I bet it's shaved and soft. It's shaved and soft, isn't it? Oh my god, you're so goddamn hot!"

Yes, this voice belonged to the self-proclaimed "King of All Media," Howard Stern. He had just debuted in LA, and I was hooked the moment he said "Show me your vagina." If you're a guy, you can't blame me. If you're a teenage guy, you know you can't help it. If you're a woman . . . I apologize.

None of the local disc jockeys flirted with strippers, talked about boobs, or described in detail the ultimate holy grail for most teenage boys: vaginas. Needless to say, I didn't make it to school on time that day because I had to see if the woman Howard was harassing was going to do it. Who was he? Who was she? What were they doing? Sex, sex, sex! That was the first of many times that I drove past the campus and skipped class so I could hear the rest of what Howard was going to say.

Perhaps my lack of academic prowess was because my parents never pressured me about my grades. As I got older, I always figured that my lack of interest was simply because I had an overactive and creative mind that just needed to be set free. Still, my dad only had three rules:

- Don't piss off your mother.
- Don't get brought home by the cops.
- When you're eighteen, you will cut your hair and get a job.

That was it . . . and in that order! He taught my brother and me many valuable lessons growing up, but these were the core three that guided my day-to-day life—especially after age ten. Moreover, his Viking-like six-foot, two-inch frame and his willingness to wield the three-foot-long spanking stick he kept in the closet was the best incentive to follow the rules. Ironically, though, I actually got decent grades, and with working around the truancy problem, I was golden when it came to *Dad Rules #1* and *#2. Yes!*

Another thing my parents never pressured me about was my weight. God bless them too, for there was plenty of pressure growing up as a fat kid in the 1980s and '90s. Why can't you run as fast as the other kids? Who are you going to take to the dance? Why don't you shower in the locker room? Why do you swim with your shirt on? Why do your nipples look like pepperonis? Can you see your own penis? Why are you so fat?

To me, growing up obese was like being buried alive. It was a prison sentence for being insecure. And at times, with normal parents and a skinny brother, it felt like a wrongful conviction that I couldn't appeal. It *sucked*, and it was one big confusing contradiction to "put on a happy face" and then have to confront the realities and ironies that came with being obese.

I remember one day in my seventh-grade English class. Mrs. Magnolia was listing our vocabulary words for the week while everybody but me took notes. I was too busy wondering if the rumor I had heard about her was true. Word on the street was that Magnolia liked a good *bammy*. She *fired up*—you know, she hit the pipe after packing it with *fresh cut grass*. I also heard that she hung out with students when tasting the herb known as the *Assassin of Youth*. Yes, Mrs. Magnolia smoked marijuana—at least, that was the word on the street.

Mrs. Magnolia wore a lot of denim (jeans and jackets). She was in her mid-forties and somewhat mousy, like a librarian. She was short too and couldn't help but get chalk dust on the back of her wrists and forearms while reaching up to write on the blackboard. With her soft and hypnotic voice, I thought of her more as a cult leader than an English teacher. As she listed our vocabulary words on the board, I pictured her in a tie-dye T-shirt and jeans with a roach clip in her chalky hand. I wasn't a pot smoker at all, but I wondered if she would rather sit in a circle, spin a Hendrix record, and smoke a bowl while reading vocabulary words. How could anyone concentrate after getting news like that?

Mrs. Magnolia broke my trance when she said, "Class, who knows what an 'oxymoron' is?"

What! What did you just call me? I thought. *"Oxy* what? Are you high right now? I shot my hand in the air and said aloud, "It's a zit cream for stupid kids, Mrs. M!"

I got a few laughs from the class, but she didn't think I was too clever. "Nooooo," she said. "Actually, an oxymoron is a noun, and I want you to memorize it for next week's spelling test. I also want you to use one in a sentence. It's a figure of speech where two words that contradict each other are used together—like *deafening silence*. Does everyone understand?"

"Oh, Mrs. M, Mrs. M . . . ," I chirped as my hand shot up and down in the air like a piston. "Or like my zit cream comment was *seriously funny*, right?"

"Right, Doug. I think you get it," she said with a twisted smile and a few brisk claps of her chalk-dusted hands.

I spent the rest of the day thinking of an oxymoron I could use in a sentence. For some reason, I thought this was the coolest thing I had learned all year. With Mrs. Magnolia reminding me more of a cult leader than a teacher, I wondered if she liked *free love*. Had she ever been told to *act naturally*? If we made a bet, would she appreciate *even odds*? And if I ditched her spelling test, would she call my parents and create a *minor crisis*?

As my mind raced, I couldn't help but feel that this oxymoron game was a little *bittersweet*. I realized that growing up fat was like an oxymoron. Maybe it was my *male sensitivity*, or maybe it was because I had always tried to be the *happy fat guy*. But I found that there was no joy in being *pleasantly plump.* In fact, being overweight as a kid, being obese, was *pretty ugly*. It was like being part of the *living dead*. And when I would think too long and too hard about how I hated being different, being obese, I often felt like a *big baby*.

I remember the first time I was outwardly upset about being overweight. I was in fifth grade and already had a beautiful set of plump man boobs. Walking home after school one day, I was obsessing about my set of boobs and matching belly. I had been sitting at my desk minutes before, tugging my shirt away from stomach every thirty seconds or so, trying to hide the fact that my belly showed through my shirt. Instead of paying attention to the teacher, I was too self-conscious about my gut. I couldn't stand how my dry T-shirt clung to my skin as if I were in a wet T-shirt contest, but in my case, there was no water. "Hey, buddy, nice tits!" was all I could think the other kids thought of me. I couldn't help but feel embarrassed.

The self-loathing I felt got worse as I continued walking home. To get to our apartment, I had to walk through the iron gates of the complex and down the long courtyard to our unit. The courtyard was narrow, like a double—or triple-wide sidewalk, and it was decorated with garden planters and little benches. Large sliding glass patio doors lined the walk as each unit opened up, opposite each other, in the courtyard. I walked past twenty units every day to get to and from our unit, as ours was on the far end.

That day, this short jaunt through the courtyard turned into a walk of shame. As I walked along, I caught sight my reflection in each sliding door. Reflection after reflection, my head would swivel to the right and to the left, trying to catch a glimpse of what I looked like. I didn't like what I saw either. I saw my belly hanging over my shorts; I looked pregnant, with boobs full of milk. I saw the profile of my butt; it looked like a beach ball full of jelly. I saw my legs; they looked like big cankles that went all the way up to my hips. I saw a kid with a sad face, and I felt disgusted.

I couldn't understand what had happened to me. I was too young to know how to deal with feeling inadequate or deep self-pity, so I asked myself aloud, "Why do you have to be so fat?" I felt normal on the inside up until then. I was a happy-go-lucky kid, and I had been skinny at one point as a younger kid. My older brother, Ben, by two years, was skinny, and I wondered, *Why isn't he fat? Why do I have to be the heavy one?* I worked myself up into a lather and got silently angry with my parents. *Why did you have to have sex and give me the fat genes? This is seriously messed up, man! I wish I had a magic wand; I would make this all disappear!*

Despite my disgust, I didn't do anything but pout. I didn't know what I could do. I was only ten and just trying to be the carefree kid I was expected to be. I never told my brother or complained to my mom and dad about being fat. They weren't around anyway. I had become a latchkey kid since moving into that apartment. Our family was in a hard spot. My mom couldn't watch me because she had to take a job as a secretary. My dad was working two shifts for minimum wage as a security guard after being asked to leave his pastor job.

I simply went inside alone and began to eat my favorite snacks, as I had been doing. There were always snacks around because my parents were buying food in bulk at the Price Club to save money. Without thinking, I binged on Pudding Pops, Pop-Tarts, and a gas tank-sized helping of soda. Feeling much better after a "light" snack, I went to ride my bike and shoot baskets at the park until my brother got home, trying to avoid the bad thoughts.

The truth of the matter is that this cycle of self-disgust and binge eating lasted for another eight or nine years. This was my struggle, appearing to be okay on the outside, happy and fun in front of people, but being seriously unhappy on the inside when I was alone. At the time, I could figure out no reason for my obesity—no violence, abuse, or bullying. However, I realized much later in life that I initially started bingeing shortly after my dad got sick. He was sent to the hospital to get well and then asked to leave our church when he got home. It was tough to see him depressed before swallowing his pride to take the security jobs. Money was tight, and I was scared that my parents would get a divorce. I thought for sure they would. All my friends' parents were getting divorces in the eighties.

What can I say? I was sensitive. I didn't know about finding personal importance or how I had stuffed my feelings, while stuffing my face, to feel some level of significance and certainty that could meet my emotional needs. It was a tough time at the Pedersen household, but it was mainly my imagination, like always, that ran things. I gained more weight, which caused me to become more insecure and mentally weak, which caused me to eat more and more—until I looked like a pumpkin with legs or the Marshmallow Man from Ghostbusters.

My poor habits didn't stop in fifth grade, even with the appearance of my man boobs. By the time I was in the ninth grade, my dad had recovered and had a stable career, and my parents were back in the community. We were in a house on the hill too, with a big pool. Still, like the bushy ivy that grew on our back fence, my shame grew deep inside my fatty shell.

That year, I was able to get my first real part-time job. *Yes! That covers Dad Rule #3. I'm golden!* I thought. As I recall, the job options were rather slim, so I worked in the cafeteria. Go figure.

Having this job was good for me, but being around the food wasn't. Everyone knows the saying about a kid in a candy store, right? Now imagine me, literally, and you can imagine the irony of the fat kid working in the school cafeteria. Of course, I worked and did what was expected of me, but I also had access to all the goodies that I shouldn't be eating. And by this age, even though I didn't know a thing about nutrition, I pretty much knew that doughnuts, pies, ice cream, and the other stuff that I was selling weren't good for me. But I couldn't resist, and instead of eating normal portions, I acted on my emotional impulses. By this point, I was a well-practiced binge eater.

I can remember seeing the other kids eat one hash brown patty after I had just eaten three or four of them. Normal kids would eat one package of snack size white powdered doughnuts when I would have two or three packages. I ate Sidewalk Sundaes and Push-Ups (ice cream), and I loved the hot apple and cherry pies that were there. Every day I would eat this stuff and more, not caring that it was sometimes cheese toast, doughnuts, pizza, and lots of chocolate milk.

Remember *Sesame Street*? How about the game they played with the song titled "One of These Things"? The game flashed a four-way split screen showing three children performing one activity, plus a fourth child "doing his own thing." Part of the song went like this: "Three of these kids belong together; three of these kids are kind of the same. But one of these kids is doing his own thing." Remember? Well, that fourth kid was me; I was "kid number four." None of the kids in school, or in the cafeteria, binged or ate in the quantities that I did. It was embarrassing and shameful. That's when I started to hide the majority of my eating and only consume when I thought no one was watching.

One of my favorite things to do was to eat apple and cherry pies during the "nutrition" break. As a cafeteria worker my job was to serve food at the snack counter and operate the cash register, but of course I never wanted to miss my *snack*. I loved the pre-wrapped pies that were shaped like half-moon pockets and filled with delightful sugary paste that never spoiled. Like a giant squirrel with a sweet tooth storing his nuts for the winter, every day I would stash one pie in the back behind the bread bin, another in the cooler box that held the milk and juices, and a third pie behind the counter underneath the cash register, to be consumed while I worked. Oh, man, it was a slick system and an efficient way to secretly eat three pies.

With a line of kids waiting to buy snacks, I could grab a bite of the pie behind the bread bin any time a kid ordered toast, a muffin, or a bagel. The same opportunity to eat more pie presented itself if a kid ordered milk or juice. I was in heaven if a kid ordered toast and milk—*Two bites, yeah!* If the line died down and there were no kids waiting, I had the pie under the counter to munch on.

As an obese youngster learning to hide his food, it was definitely *bittersweet*. I knew that I looked like a pig, and I was self-conscious about eating so many pies and everything else I managed to get from the cafeteria. Still, around the other kids I tried to act as if being heavy didn't bother me. I just tried to play it off a lot in public and act cool. Never let them see you sweat, you know? I believed that this was who I was, and that I was destined to be a guilty food sneaker whom everyone liked. If I had only known or had the maturity to understand that I was choosing the worst possible (negative) way to feel and meet my emotional needs.

There were times when I tried to do something about losing weight and fought back. Usually, though, my partially completed attempts at starting a diet or trying to exercise were more like throwing a Hail Mary pass in football, a last-ditch effort. I made them make-or-break situations. My attempts were obsessive impulses that had absolutely no chance of lasting or getting me any real results. It didn't help that my shame and pride kept me from asking for help—from my parents, from a teacher, from a coach, or from anybody. I acted like such a smart-ass all the time; how could anyone know that I was dying on the inside?

During Christmas of 1985, I asked my parents for exercise equipment. Thankfully, they put a good word in with Santa (*wink*). I found two five-pound dumbbells waiting for me under the tinsel my mom had shaped like a tree on our living room curtains that year. I had no idea how to exercise, but I knew that I didn't want to be fat. These dumbbells were my saving grace, and I thought of them as my own magic wand (pathetic, I know). With one lift of a weight, I dreamed that they would help shrink my belly or make my boobs disappear. Or if I held them in each hand and bent over, I prayed that my butt might actually become a normal size. To no avail. These weights—these tiny gifts from heaven that acted more like shiny door stoppers than a pair of magic wands—came in handy when I would feel at my lowest, desperate and sick about my weight.

You can do this, Doug, I would say to myself. *I bet if you do fifty curls right now, your biceps will pop out like Arnold Schwarzenegger's instead of hanging like the limp sausage arms John Candy sports. Go for it!* I would huff and puff and imagine that I was really getting a tough workout—even though the five-pounders didn't offer much resistance. I don't think that I even worked up a sweat or turned my skin the reddish flushed color you get when you've exerted your muscles or your lungs. But I was young and greatly wanted to change my appearance. I'd get my fifty reps and then look down at my bicep to check for a muscle. I would even look at my stomach and see if it got smaller. Sometimes I would flex my knee and see if my leg felt any different.

This was totally obsessive, desperate, and insane—but the equation worked in my imagination. More than anything else, I just wanted to have a magic wand and make my belly disappear. I wanted to wake up one day to Doug. I wanted to go back to when I was four, five, or six: "normal" and "skinny." What happened to that guy? What was my problem?

Without fail, I would run to the mirror and check myself out, only to see that my face was now long—like the kid who got a math book for Christmas instead of a BB gun. I couldn't help but get disgusted and defeated. Of course, my body didn't change a bit, but I wanted it so bad. I tried things like this all the time, which always made me feel helpless. As a kid, I didn't know what more I could do, if anything. I felt trapped; I felt buried alive without any help; I felt like a failure.

Another classic episode involved my trips to the grocery store. One time in high school, I went snack shopping on a Saturday morning because I was so bored. I checked out all the usual stuff—candy, ice cream, the deli counter, the bakery—and somehow I ended up in the diet aisle. I stood there mesmerized because I had been obsessing over Slim-Fast and Dexatrim commercials for a while, over their diet pills that promised to help you lose weight in a jiff. I wanted it so much, to just take a pill and drop the pounds. I wanted to believe that it was that easy to melt the fat away. I must have stood in that aisle for twenty minutes, reading the box, looking around, waiting for people to empty the aisles so that I could sneak my *fat secret* up to the register.

For some reason, I was embarrassed to be a fat kid buying diet pills in public. It was crazy. Everybody could see that I was heavy and probably didn't even care, but I just couldn't bring myself to buy them. I imagined the cashier looking at the box as she scanned my items, stopping a moment to look at me and then rolling her eyes before mumbling "That figures" to herself. What if she didn't chastise me but asked for my ID? You had to be eighteen to purchase diet pills (legal speed, woo-hoo!) What if I went for it and the people behind me saw as I held up the line. I couldn't handle it if they all looked over at me and muttered, "Huh? A fat kid's buying diet pills. That figures!"

I couldn't bring myself to make the purchase. Instead, I waddled directly to the freezer aisle and grabbed a half gallon of chocolate chip ice cream. For some reason, "the fat kid buying ice cream" was more acceptable to me than "the fat kid buying diet pills." I figured that people expected that, and so did I. That day I went home and ate that whole carton in one sitting, like a dog that hadn't eaten for weeks. No one else was home, so I parked my butt on the couch and I killed it. Judging by the pace that I kept, you would've thought that there was a diamond waiting for me at the bottom of the carton. Bite after bite, I just kept shoveling ice cream in my mouth until it was gone. My tongue was frozen and the brain freeze crept up my nose, but I didn't care, nor did I let it phase me. I was too busy sucking the cream down my throat and then chewing the mouth full of hard chocolate chips that were left behind. Who had time for brain freezes? I was feeling good!

In a twist that not even I expected, I cracked my goddamned tooth on the very last bite. True story. *What the fudge (cicle)?* I thought. I spit out a chunk of molar that rivaled the diamond that wasn't waiting for me at the bottom of the carton. I was shocked, to say the least. I couldn't believe that I broke a tooth on ice cream! *Isn't this a bitch,* I thought. *Who would believe this one?* "Hey, did you hear the one about the kid in Burbank? Yeah, he ate so much ice cream one day that he actually died on his couch. Turns out, he choked on his own tooth! Somewhere in the melee a molar popped out and got stuck in his pie hole. Yeah. The doctors got there too late, but they managed to defrost his brain before the funeral. Did you see it? It was sponsored by Chips Ahoy!"

I couldn't believe it. I was pissed, embarrassed, and ashamed all at the same time. How could I tell my parents that I broke my tooth while eating ice cream on a Saturday morning? So I didn't tell a soul, and I didn't do anything about the break. I tried to ignore it, like everything else that made me unhappy. Looking back, this wasn't the smartest thing I've ever done. Had I known that my cracked tooth would become infected, I would've clearly told my parents a lie! But I didn't do anything, so sure enough I got a tooth infection and a nice root canal to go with it. Wow. How stupid and even more insignificant I felt after that. The bridge that's in my mouth to this day is a nice reminder of how *good* that ice cream was. *Crap, and no diamond!*

Failing in private was bad enough; failing in front of other people was horrifying. I learned this when I was finally old enough to play high school sports. I let this turn out to be a real disaster for me too because I was scared to put myself out there and compete. But my brother, Ben, had played two years of junior varsity football and was trying out for the varsity team. Ben was always popular and was well liked by the other guys, the girls, and the coaches. He was the starting center on the offensive line, and he had some intimidating stories of hitting pads in practice, lifting weights, or laying hits on the other team during the games. It sounded tough: practice, games, hitting, showering with guys, weight lifting . . . It all intimidated me.

Needless to say, being a 240-pound freshman and the brother of a starting varsity offensive lineman, the coaches were excited to see me try out. I also thought that my dad really wanted me to go for it because although he always wanted to play, he had to stay and work the farm with his brothers and sisters. He didn't pressure me, but I pressured myself. I still felt as if he expected me to play—to be tough like him and like

Ben—and I thought that playing high school football was necessary to earn his pride.

I remember the first day of tryouts. Everything seemed all right until the coach blew his whistle and bellowed, "Okay, boys! We're going to start with some agility drills and work into the tryout. Big boys on the right. Pedersen! That's you. Eyes here, son; you need to pay attention. Get over there with the other lineman. We're going to make you into a feared run blocker!"

"What did he just say?" I mumbled to myself. "Agility drills; is he serious? I hope not, because I'm agile like an elephant, like a hibernating bear, or maybe more like the couch I left to come here today." While I moped over to "the right," I told a buddy, "Feared run blocker? I'm more like an artery blocker; know what I mean?"

With a blow of the coach's whistle, the practice intensified like a forest fire. Guys were yelling as the coaches ran us through the pad sled drills. We did push-up drills, laps, and wind sprints. I did my first sprint, which looked more like a giant hopping baby, and I could feel my butt swing violently up and down like a tugboat in a monsoon. "Let's go, Pedersen. Move that big body, son!" I heard repeatedly.

FU, Coach! It was horrible.

They quickly moved us to the burpee drills, which I also hated. Burpees were evil to slow, fat guys like me, and unfortunately I couldn't make them go away with Gasex. I thought you needed to be a gymnast to do a burpee correctly; I was more like a sumo wrestler. Anyway, the burpee movement called for us to quickly bend down and put our hands on the ground (yeah, right), kick our legs back (*kick*? not a chance), do a push-up (in my case, maybe one), bring our legs back in, and stand up (I could stand). We were to do that as many times as we could in a minute or so. I didn't do any of them right. I could bend down partly, but there was no way I could do the rest, or at least that's what I told myself. I mimicked everything and tried to look like I was putting in some effort while the other guys just grunted them out.

We hit the pad sled next. The coach placed the squad in a line in three-point stances. He blew his damn whistle and told us to explode into the pads and then drive (push) the sled across the field.

Yeah, right! I thought. *I would rather "explode" in my pants right about now.* Needless to say, I exploded into that pad sled with the power of a baby chicken. I was on the end too, and it hardly moved. The other guys pushed so hard that the sled almost did a full 180-degree turn.

"Come on, Pedersen! Drive those legs!" I heard.

Drive this, ass wipe! I mean, Coach.

With my dainty ego firmly in check, I prepared for the monkey drills. *Great, finally something I can do. Yeah, right!* In this drill, three guys would lay on the ground facing down, in a push-up position. When the coach blew the whistle, the three guys were expected to alternate pushing up and bouncing over each other, landing back in the push up-position—and do it as fast as they could. It basically looked like how a juggler juggles three balls, except every guy had to time his own bounce to avoid getting landed on. Let's just say that this was a complete nightmare for me. I got in the mix and was rolled on, bounced on, and creamed by guys stronger and way more agile than I. In the end, it must've looked like a game of "dog pile on Doug."

I was done after that; I couldn't take it anymore. I was so embarrassed and defeated. I didn't want to be there, so I quit. I kept telling myself through the whole tryout, which for me couldn't have lasted more than thirty minutes, that I was too fat, that I wasn't agile or fast, that I couldn't do push-ups or run, and that I couldn't bounce from the ground to my feet or do anything. Like many other things, I believed that I wasn't good enough. So after the first set of monkey drills, I walked to the back of the line, and when nobody was looking, I simply turned and left the field. I didn't tell anybody at all, none of the guys or the coaches. How could I? I felt humiliated and pathetic. I was broken and felt as if I let the coaches break me, and even then, I knew that the truth was that I had broken myself. The worst part meant facing my brother and my dad at some point. I didn't know how I was going to tell them that I quit. What was I going to say? I was a real mess.

I felt worthless, and I might have even cried on the way home. I was sure that my dad and my brother would be able to see right through me—my fear and my pathetic, fat, weak-minded self. How could I face them? My dad was so strong-minded and physical, battling his own way, and my older brother was exactly like him. Here I was—the one who was different and couldn't hack it. I wanted to run away. Instead, I just ate more, and I was too young and inexperienced in life to know how this simple pattern actually, and exactly, satisfied my most important emotional needs at a very high level.

Despite my poor performance with the drills, the head coach actually called me at home the next day and encouraged me to play. That's how desperate they were. I wrestled with it for a few days, and my dad didn't say much (which might have been the worst of all), but I eventually swallowed my pride and went back to the field and tried to compete. They put me on the offensive line, and I played center, the guy who hikes the ball to the quarterback, like Ben did. I wasn't good or fast, and I looked like Dumpy Smurf in the powder-blue football pants we wore. Oh, how my love handles hung out over the hip pads like pork roasts. We were awful too, like the Bad News Bears of high school football, and we couldn't do anything right during the practices or during the games. We lost all eleven games that year, and all our coaches were fired.

I quit sports for good after that. It was easy not to go back for a second season after losing so much. I could blame the team for not wanting to play again. It was great because I was able to stop playing and save some face with my friends. No one had to know that I quit on myself. So that was it. I traded in the practice pads for a part-time job. I tried to keep my image as a cool, nice guy, but I had lost all confidence in myself. And having quit the only physically challenging thing I had done in a few years, I was sure that I was going to weigh five hundred pounds eventually. Why not? I ate whatever I wanted, and I hated to run and do anything physical. It was too hard and too embarrassing. I didn't know how to build my confidence again or feel the positive side of self-importance (significance), so I was sure that I was on the road to doubling my weight someday. Gaining weight was the only sure thing at which I wouldn't fail.

After quitting football, I had plenty of time for other emotions beyond shame and failure—the worst of them all was "comfort." Comfort was the worst emotion because feeling comfortable about my obesity meant that I had accepted it as my version of "normal." It meant that carrying around over one hundred extra pounds on my body was okay. How could carrying the fat equivalent of a baby deer around my waist be okay? It meant that having a huge belly and man boobs was okay. It meant that binge eating was my fate. Comfort meant that there was no turning back to ever being skinny again; no trying to change or fix my problems anymore; no hope for a normal life with a normal girlfriend or a normal job. *At least I didn't quit on my man boobs,* I would sadly joke to myself.

Without football, I also had time to get a better job. That's when I made my next big career move and got hired pumping gas. I didn't mind the dirty job, and I didn't mind my colorful coworkers. But I didn't much care for the fact that I became the "butt" of many jokes. No, seriously—my butt became the joke. I heard so much about it that I thought the mechanics had the specs to my butt crack in their car manuals.

Ron was the ringleader. He was a tall strapping guy with a big bushy mustache and small slits for eyes. He was only twenty-four or twenty-five, but at the time, he was a real adult to me. Ron was also a bit of a redneck (pardon the stereotype), and I always wondered how he ended up in LA, with his flattop hair, a jacked-up four-by-four truck, and a Southern accent. He also was obviously fascinated with my butt crack.

"Jesus, Doug!" Ron would shout from across the garage. "I can see your butt crack all the way from here. Are you sure you got your shirt tucked in? Damn, son! You're butt crack is bigger than the Rio Grande!"

Ron said this to me nearly every day. It didn't bother me so much at first, but I heard it so many times that I actually had to look up "Rio Grande." And once I figured out that he thought my butt crack was bigger than the river that separates the United States and Mexico, I could hardly disagree with him. Let's face facts; at the time (and even to this day, folks), I had a large butt crack. It was so large and so long that it reached halfway up my back—or so I felt much of the time. In addition to its *grande* stature, it didn't help me with Ron or with the other guys, considering the fact that my uniform shirts didn't stay tucked in, giving my massive crack the opportunity to make an appearance most of the time I labored around the station.

The other guys eventually picked on up the joke with Ron. Because I didn't defend myself, I suppose they found it easy to. Sam was an older guy who picked up every coin he ever saw on the ground. The guys messed with him by gluing pennies to the concrete. Sam messed with me by constantly trying to check my butt crack's pressure like a tire. It was a little weird. But so was Sam, and it made the other guys laugh hysterically.

25

Art was the best because he actually showed me how to do things. He taught me how to fix a tire and change the oil in a car. When Art wasn't teaching me, he was trying to lodge things in my butt crack. Nothing dangerous, but he would launch popcorn, wing nuts, and valve stems in my crack's general direction all the time. One time he got really crazy and lobbed an air filter at it. For those who don't know, an air filter looks like a doughnut and is the size of a record. He threw a soft underhand pitch, and it glanced on my butt cheek without an issue, but that got the garage going. Ron thought it was the funniest. "Shee-iitt! Can you imagine if that filter lodged in there? I think it had a chance too. That's funny, Arty!"

If only someone knew that I was stuffing my face, stuffing my emotions, in order to feel some level of significance and certainty in my life . . . I was an oxymoron; I was ashamed; I felt like a failure; I was the guy who was the ultimate butt crack of all jokes (not to mention the owner of a great set of tits).

CHAPTER 3

CUT YOUR HAIR AND GET A JOB

Chances multiply when you take them.
—Doug Pedersen

Have you ever made a simple choice that had huge consequences? You know, ever made a choice that seemed small, but its meaning grew like a snowball rolling down a mountain? Not like choosing a mate or choosing to go after your first thirty-year adjustable-rate mortgage—yikes! I'm talking about a no-brainer, a no-big-deal decision—the kind of choice you make when you're seventeen. But somehow, when you weren't looking, and maybe only when you really stopped to think about it, that small choice actually changed your life. This happened to me when I chose to follow *Dad Rule #3* and become a security guard.

Like I mentioned in the previous chapter, *Dad Rule #3* required that my brother and I have legitimate jobs by the age of eighteen. The rule didn't say what kind of work we had to do. The rule simply stated that we needed to be presentable in public and support ourselves someday. Actually, to quote the man, it went more like this: "Boys, the free ride will be over soon. Don't kid yourself about living under my roof for free with your mother and me. You *will* be weaned from the teat! When you're eighteen, you need to cut your hair and get a job."

My brother, Ben, and I heard "When you're eighteen, cut your hair and get a job" starting at a very early age. This wasn't a scare tactic from an overbearing dad. It was actually said out of love in an instructive way, like "Here's your roadmap to becoming a man." In fact, my dad started teaching us the value of honest work maybe even before I spoke English. "Ha-ha-ha. He said *teat*," the two-year-old chuckled while skimming the classifieds.

My dad's name is Bill, and he's awesome. There's no doubt that he's my hero, and I love him very much. He's a real provider, a protector, and a family man. Bill is also the epitome of a man's man, a real straight shooter with a get-it-done type of attitude. You won't find a more honest person than him, and he is the guy whom people love to have in charge.

A mountain of a man (literally), my dad has hands like a polar bear. His shoulders are broad, and his neck and wrists are thick, like a wrestler's. He's not a big football fan, but he has been called "Hey, Ditka!" in public before, if you get my drift. Dad's *city* now, but I always figured that *Dad Rule #3* came from his more rural roots. See, Bill grew up doing manual labor on the Nebraska farm where he and his nine brothers and sisters were raised, which also gave him an amazing work ethic and a most genuine heart. It apparently also gave him amazing insight into *teat weaning*.

Dad had other quotable moments besides *Dad Rules*. When he wasn't busy working, Ben and I could often talk him into taking us to the neighborhood pool. But not before we heard, "You boys are too *city*; your uncle Carl and I used to swim in irrigation ditches." Or if we wanted to watch a show like *The Love Boat* or *Alf*, he would say, "You boys are too *city*; whatever happened to *The Rifleman* or *The Lone Ranger*?" He's absolutely right, though. I'm a city boy through and through, and I liked Los Angeles. The only thing I've ever done in an irrigation ditch is take a leak during a family reunion.

I didn't think that it got too cold in Burbank, California. Still, sometimes Dad liked to say, "It's colder than a coaly's ass in here!" Or if we were at the beach he'd say, "Watch your nuts, boys. That water is colder than a coaly's ass." I didn't understand the *coaly* reference until much later. It actually took me thirty years to figure out that he was relating the temperature to a guy's butt—or more specifically, a coal miner's butt. A coaly (a coal miner, I think) whose butt must get very cold while working underground. That's obvious, right?

Even though Dad was an ordained minister at one point, he still would commit blasphemy. "Jesus Christ, Anne! The boy is five years old," he would tell my mother while defending his decision to let Ben and me launch ourselves off the high dive. Or, "Jesus Christ, Anne! The boy is nine. It didn't even come close to his toes," he said, before snatching the electric chain saw from my hands as we worked in the yard. "Jesus Christ, Anne! The boy is seventeen. Of course he'll graduate; he'll only be sitting behind a desk passing out radios to the other security guards."

My mom really had nothing to worry about. Dad's the pragmatic type, and he never would have let anything happen to us. Plus, I never aspired to be a real super trooper. At the time, I only knew two things about security work: everybody dressed like Andy Griffith, and Dad had worked as a security guard when I was a younger kid. It was during the rough patch in the mid-1980s, as I mentioned before. He was searching for work after leaving our church, and he took security shifts that paid $4.11 per hour. He used to tell my brother and me, "*Four eleven* is better than *no eleven*. And if you get two *four elevens*, that's *eight twenty-two*. You do what you have to do, boys." To this day, my dad still uses the "four eleven" speech when referring to work, or anything in life, that isn't particularly fun. Like a mantra for getting through things that suck.

I never forgot my dad's ability to focus on a task and do whatever was necessary. When my task was to stop going to high school during my senior year, I remembered *Dad Rule #3*. Working was the perfect *out* from class. Why not work more, get paid more, and get away from the mechanics at the gas station who played basketball with my backside? So I applied to a work experience program and got it. My guidance counselor only required that I keep my B average and enroll in the college-level English and math courses. My reaction: "*Whatever!*" But I did what she said and then asked my dad to help me get a job as a guard. You can imagine my excitement when they wanted to pay me *nine fifty-five*. Wow! One *nine fifty-five* crushes two *four elevens*.

Now to bring the story full circle, this simple choice started an enormous series of snowballing events. I didn't realize it at the time, nor was I looking for it, but working security at Universal Studios Hollywood changed my life forever. It was huge, like a divine intervention. I had taken this job for superficial reasons as a chump teenager. No long-term perspective here; just a kid looking to get out of class and earn some easy money for babysitting something. However, two powerful miracles happened while I tried to float through this job: I met "Lovable Louie," who helped me find ambition, and I lost a few fluke pounds for the first time ever.

The fix was in with my new security job. There wasn't really much of an application or screening process, especially with my dad vouching for me. He had made quite a name for himself coming up through the security ranks at Universal Studios (a.k.a. "Universal" or just "the Studios"). By the time I stumbled in at Universal in the winter of 1991, he was the chief of investigations for corporate security and was sort of a bigwig.

Universal is a massive group of TV and movie-making studios that also runs a theme park for tourists. It's situated in North Hollywood on a 480-acre property only a few miles from where I grew up. Shows like *Magnum P.I., The A-Team, Knight Rider,* and *Bonanza* were produced there. Movies like *ET, Back to the Future,* and *Jurassic Park* were huge there. The theme park is open to the public—after you buy a ticket, of course—and attracts close to twenty thousand tourists a day from all over the world. I was excited to work there because, like many kids in the eighties, I had grown to be a huge fan of TV and movies; I had grown up to be a huge couch potato. Even a local kid like me was struck by the magic of Hollywood when I got to see famous people like Jean-Claude Van Dame, Bob Hope, and even Michael Jackson in person.

Through a stroke of luck, I got the best job on the shift. Actually, my dad pulled some strings and they put me in the main security office of the theme park. It was called "Tours Security," and I was the swing shift dispatcher. I laughed out loud when I heard what my job was. My main responsibilities included passing out radios, answering phones, recording alarms, dispatching the roving guards, and coordinating their breaks. To me, this translated into sit on your butt, sit on your butt some more, visit the Riverboat food stand and grab some hot dogs, sit on your butt again, take a dump, and finally go back to the desk and sit on your butt until your shift is over. I thought it was the perfect job for a kid with my type of ambition—with the ambition of a throw pillow.

Being the dispatcher didn't only involve desk work. There was some light walking involved too. On top of dispatching guards, they also wanted me to watch the front door and greet the tourists that approached our office. The door was cut in half—like the door to a day-care playroom—and seemed like it was a mile away. Actually, it was only six whole feet from my desk, which just made it a pain in the ass anytime someone stopped by. Some tourists tried to open our "cubby door" to come in, so I was supposed to greet them and find out "what the fucking problem was." Most of them wanted to know where to find *Conan the Barbarian*, the *Miami Vice* set, or the famous gray DeLorean from *Back to the Future*, which they literally had to walk by to get to our door. A lot of them also thought that our office was the bathroom. One time a guy tried the doorknob for what seemed like thirty seconds, kicking the door while looking at me and my boss before saying, "Are you going to let me in or what? I'm about to shit my pants out here in front of my little girl!"

"Calm down, sir, and step away from the little girl right now!" was all I could think to say.

It was a fun job, and I encountered many interesting people. Working with the other guards brought lots of goofy situations similar to the movies *Armed and Dangerous*, *Paul Blart: Mall Cop*, and *Super Troopers*. The tourists were great too, but you had to watch out for little nuances like the kamikaze tourists who didn't pay attention to where they walked or the pooping dad that used his daughter as a human shield. Most security incidents were minor as well. The park quieted down after seven o'clock at night, and then it was about locking the place down and keeping an eye on things—a good time for mischief between the guards and the other park employees.

My favorite caper was raiding the food kitchens for leftovers. Restaurants like the Italian Kitchen or The Park Grille were great for getting big plates of pasta, pizza, and soda. Another of my favorite food scores was the Riverboat. It was a patio-style concession counter that looked like it was steaming down the mighty Mississippi—big waterwheel and all. I've already documented my bingeing habits, so there's no need to revisit them. But you can imagine my delight while smelling many freshly wrapped warm hot dogs that had been tossed in the garbage that night. Yes, I had no shame then either.

As dispatcher, I got to spend a lot of time with a guy I chose to admire more than a Riverboat hot dog: Lovable Louie. Louie was a manager, and to me he was the most interesting guy in the room. Our desks sat facing each other, and I worked the radio while he called the shots. He was in his early sixties and wore a full head of silver hair that he combed straight back—like Pat Riley. Louie's eyes were always wide open, watching everything, and although he was polished, he had a rough, manly look illustrated best by the pear-size tattoo on his right forearm. The ink was dark green and faded; you could tell that it had been there a while.

I thought Louie's background was fascinating from the very beginning. He was retired from the Los Angeles Police Department (LAPD). If you brought it up, which I often did, he would let you know that he had done and seen everything. He worked homicide and vice; he worked police Intel and covered organized crime; he was a detective and had investigated some of LA's most famous crimes and murders. Louie also was a member of the elite Special Investigative Service (SIS) at one point. SIS was notorious for taking down big criminals, the worst of the worst. They were even more high speed and ruthless than SWAT.

Before running the streets for thirty years with LAPD, Louie was a United States Marine. He enlisted after the Korean War and did his own time during the Vietnam War, in the late 1950s and '60s. That's when he got the tattoo on his forearm of the Marine's famous insignia: the eagle, globe, and anchor. As a Marine, Louie was a grunt, an infantryman, and a sniper. Although he didn't like to talk about his experiences in Vietnam, he was a wealth of knowledge when it came to Marine Corps history, World War II trivia, and on life in the Corps. You knew that Louie was proud of the Marines and happy to greet other veterans that joined the security team. "Semper Fi! Once a Marine always a Marine!" he would bark out across the office.

Louie was also a crafty flirt. That's how he got the nickname "Lovable Louie." He always amazed me with his effortless charm. I'm not saying that he was a ladies' man, because Louie had a ton of respect for women, especially his wife. But he was a widower, and I could tell that he liked the feeling when he would flirt a little and get some playful admiration, and even some validation, in return. Louie had what I called the "Harry Connick Junior effect." He didn't say anything to be especially funny or outwardly flirty. It was more his aura—just his energy, I suppose. Still, the women giggled at everything he said. He could say, "These cherries are amazing! I love the chocolate-covered cherries that come from Michigan in the fall. Aren't they lovely? They remind me of a cute bed-and-breakfast where you can sleep in and take long romantic walks among the foliage." Every female security guard would melt and start to giggle. "Oh, Louie, you're just so gosh darn lovable!"

Oh, Louie, you're such a sly devil, I would think to myself as he winked at me. For a native Angelino, he reminded me of a European ladies' man, with a slight raspy voice from smoking too many cigarettes. I always waited for him to follow up with a cheesy line like, "Tell me something, doll; if I told you that you had an amazing body, would you hold it against me?" But he never did.

Louie was the type of guy that you wanted next to you in the foxhole. You wanted to be on his team. He was the warrior poet type: strong yet sensitive and foul-mouthed in private yet eloquent in public. He was the guy you were sort of afraid to make mad but who could make you laugh out loud. "Doug!" he once said. "Who was that—that fucking guard with the short pants? Was he serious with those maroon socks? Call his ass back in here." When the guy showed up, Louie stood up, planted his foot on top of the desk, and pulled his own pant leg up. "Blue or black—not fucking maroon! Now go get some new goddamned socks before Doug's dad sees you!" he scolded while pointing at his dark blue socks. The guy looked at me while his ass puckered like a lime tart before darting out the door. "How'd I do, Doug?" he'd say with a grin.

Louie took me under his wing. He showed me what to do and helped me get respect from the other guards. Instead of being around younger greasy mechanics who razzed me about my butt crack, I was now working under a guy who showed me respect—and I respected him. I figured that he did this out of respect for my dad because they were friends. But later on, I felt that Louie did this out of respect for me. "Doug!" he would say. "You're a good man. You've earned your salt. Your dad was right about you." I didn't know what he meant at the time, but I knew that it just felt good to be respected, to feel a bit of confidence and self-esteem. Admiring Louie struck me like a magic trick after I had spent so much time floating through school and avoiding responsibility. It was inspiring; it was like being mentored in a way that parents can't—like when you're seventeen and think you know everything already. It was valuable, and it was the beginning of some very big changes in my life.

In time, Louie trusted me to make decisions for the shift. He preferred to be out of the office making rounds anyway, versus sitting in the office processing paperwork. Once he felt that I could handle it, Louie would leave the office like a thief in the night and disappear for hours on end. The office to him was like school for me. There were times where I would see him maybe once in an eight-hour shift. We talked on the radio or on the phone a lot, but he hated the office. Without fail, though, Louie would stroll in thirty minutes before shift change and say, "Doug! What happed today?" as he walked through the door. It was like his announcement that he was there. "Doug! What happed today?" meant "Hey, Doug. How are ya? Tell me what I need to tell the oncoming shift so that we can get the hell outta here!" I would run down the list of events and always get cut off: "Doug! Did we get reports for all that?" The answer was always yes, and he would say, "You're a good man, Doug. Your dad was right about you. Enough nonsense—now let's go get an ice cream."

Louie always had a backup watch the radio, and we'd walk and talk about stuff while we ate ice cream together. I really got the sense that he liked me, and I used that opportunity to ask him about everything. And I listened to every story Louie would tell about his life as a cop and as a Marine.

Almost a year into my time with Louie, the Studio hosted a huge special event called "Halloween Horror Nights." It was October 1992, and I had graduated high school a few months before, in June. The event lasted the entire month, and it sure lived up to its name. The park transformed into a huge haunted house full of ghosts, goblins, werewolves, and witches that shrieked in horror. Fog machines blanketed the park with thick wet smoke, and miles of fake cobwebs, loud bloodcurdling sound effects, and frightened tourists filled the park. The first time I walked to the office at night, I thought that even Count Dracula might crap his pants if he saw this setup.

The park hours also extended to 9 p.m. and the attendance increased from twenty thousand people per day to almost forty or fifty thousand. For us, that meant more incidents and more guards to watch everything. The surge in coverage also meant that the shift needed an additional supervisor. The new supervisor was supposed to make sure that all the others were where they needed to be when they were supposed to be there—or so I thought.

Much to my surprise, Louie asked me to be his junior field supervisor for the month. I never asked him for it because I thought I was a long shot as the youngest guy on the shift, and I felt honored that he considered me. I wondered if he was just trying to stay on my dad's good side, but I wanted to please him anyway. Louie had other concerns besides maroon socks, and he refused to let anything big happen on his watch. As a result, he told me to check the guards at least three times per shift. Wanting to do a good job, my plan was to check everybody at least five times—walking from post to post and checking socks and haircuts, also being the first responder if an incident happened. When I wasn't doing that, I thought I could catch some of the shows. "Don't get any smart ideas, Doug. I need you in the parking lots; you're going to be *Lord of the Lots*—get it? I need someone out there that I can trust to keep those slappers in line. It's going to be busy, Doug, so buckle up."

I didn't know if "slappers" were the tourists or the guards. Turned out Louie was referring to the other guards, like *slap dicks* or just plain *slappers*. It's a cop thing, I guess, but I understood what he meant after my first shift. I thought he should have called me *King of the Dipshits* instead of *Lord of the Lots* because the new parking lot guards followed directions as well as a rogue vampire.

My first shift set the tone for an action-packed month. And as Louie had told me, it was busier than a Chinese train station at high noon. I made an activity plan (for the first time ever) and set my sights on getting around to all the guards five times minimum, thinking that should take up the entire shift. With my clipboard in hand, I was "on the beat" for the first four hours (from 3 p.m. to 7 p.m.), checking guards posted in the parking garages and in the many parking lots. I walked a lot but was also able to hitch rides on golf carts here and there. But like a sudden thunder and lightning strike—or the moment in a college party where the alcohol seems to hit everyone at the same time—at 7 p.m. the shift instantly went from dull to *what the hell*!

"Zombie down! Zombie down!" was the radio call that changed everything. Once this hit the security airwaves, I was running like Forrest Gump—or at least trying to—because incident after incident tore through the park. The "zombie call" turned out to be funnier than the panicked voice on the radio let on. Once I got there, I saw that a tourist from Amsterdam had literally flattened an actor that was in character as a zombie in the Horror Maze. Apparently, the actor jumped out of the wall and scared the poop out of our friend from Amsterdam. The Dutchman didn't appreciate that one bit and felt that a punch in the face was a fair trade for a poop in the pants.

Before I could clear that scene, I got another hair-raising call. "My foot! My foot! This is post forty-nine, and I've just been run over by a yellow taxi!" Turns out the guard's foot didn't get run over. But he did have an altercation where the cab driver opened his car door into the guard. You know, like the guard was standing too close to the car and got bumped when the guy opened his door. There were no major injuries—or injuries, period—but I still had to call the paramedics, get all the operations managers involved, and get statements from all fifty witnesses who saw our guy basically provoke the whole thing. Whoopsie!

The next significant incident involved a man and a horse. Actually, the radio call went like this: "Dope in the turnstiles! I've got dope in the turnstiles!" I learned when I arrived on the scene that our guard thought he saw somebody trying to sell marijuana to the tourists. All I saw was a guy passing out brochures, inappropriately of course, but I didn't see any reefer bags. Then I saw a West Hollywood sheriff deputy in full gallop, coming straight toward me on horseback. The sheriffs were on the property for serious incidents, and this cop thought we were serious. He was serious at least. He wore tall black leather riding boots to the knee and had a riot stick that was as long as a samurai sword. His olive-green cowboy hat covered the biggest handlebar mustache I'd ever seen. The horse skid in front of me while the sheriff grunted, "Where is he?" I pointed in the general direction of the brochure guy while the officer dismounted. "Here, hold my horse!" He passed me the reins and smartly stepped to the perp. I stood there in amazement, eye-to-eye with a horse that was huffing and puffing in my face—the snot literally dripped from both its nostrils. *I'm too city, eh? If Dad could only see me now*, I thought.

I had to pick up the pieces after all those incidents. It was my job to coordinate the scene, getting the right operations managers, paramedics, and cops to deal with the melee. It was my job to respond, assess, take control, and then gather the information before writing reports for the security bosses—for Louie. Smaller incidents always popped up in between the big ones, like a lost child or a tourist that couldn't remember which of the ten parking lots he'd parked his rental car in. Every day that month was like that, and I thought it was exciting. It was like being in a TV show versus watching a TV show. So much drama; so much to talk about; so little time to think about anything, especially eating or drowning in any type of self-loathing thoughts.

By the end of the event, I had earned my own little reputation, at least with Louie. "Doug! You were definitely *Lord of the Lots*. They should name a character after you." I didn't know how to take his praise. I just thought I was doing my job, and I wanted to please him. But I think Louie sensed that I wanted more. He could see that I was thriving in the role and had become more confident with the other guards. That's when he said, "Doug! You're a good man, and you did a good job for me. I want to promote you permanently. Do you think you can handle it?"

I wanted to keep that job more than anything. I felt I had succeeded at something, and I knew I was capable of more; maybe I could run the shift at some point. I'd never had ambitions like that before. Usually I was trying to find the easier route, and I could've easily snuck back into the office as his dispatcher. When I asked him what my job would be, he simply said, "I'm going to make some changes when these slappers leave. You're going to be second in charge, after me. I tell you what to do, and then you tell them what to do. Get it? Do you think you can handle that?" I was ecstatic and still a little surprised. I was the youngest guy on the shift and thought that others would think I got promoted because of my dad. For the first time in a long time, though, I dismissed what others might think. I told Louie, "Hell yeah!"

"Good, but get your uniforms switched out over the weekend. You look like hell, man! We don't want people thinking you're the *Sultan of Slappers*."

Louie was right; I looked like hell. In the end, Halloween Horror Nights turned out to be my "sweaty lip month." You know, how you're upper lip glistens with small beads of sweat. No? Just me? Well, as a 275-pound eighteen-year-old racing around a 480-acre fun house, my upper lip was never dry. My collar was never clean, always soiled from the ring around the collar, and my pits were always steamy. I was a busy beaver, and I worked (walked) my ass off. As a result, I wore a sweat mustache on my upper lip most of the time.

I knew that my uniforms fit differently before Louie mentioned it. I never analyzed it, though, because I didn't have the time. When I got home that night, I stepped on my parents' scale and couldn't believe my eyes. By the time it registered my weight, the digital screen read 250.

"Wow—250 pounds? Me?" I hadn't weighed 250 since the tenth grade. I leaped off the scale with joy and looked in the mirror. I hadn't seen a smile that big since I got dumbbells for Christmas. I was amazed that during the four weeks of Halloween Horror Nights, I lost twenty-five pounds without trying. It was shocking, and it blew my mind. I stood there in disbelief, just letting the wonder run through my mind. Not only had I never had sex before; I had never lost weight before—ever! My steady weight gains as a kid didn't allow me to believe that any of this was even possible. This was a miracle, a divine intervention, my first victory in my heavyweight bout with obesity—and it felt as if I had dominated the first round.

The reality of this important victory was due to the fact that I was cut off from eating so much junk food—because I didn't have access to the Riverboat—and went from a stationary post behind a desk to a roving post where I was in a constant state of movement. Very slow movement too. Sure, I made it into the park to get some food here and there, but nothing like what I had been doing before. And as a young teenager, I never packed my lunch and I never planned. My plan had always been to get something, a lot of something, for free—or to just buy a pizza when that didn't work out. But during the Halloween Horror Nights, I simply didn't have the time. I was too busy going from guard to guard. I wanted to please my bosses and do a good job, so I didn't take breaks. As a result, I avoided a lot of soda, tons of hot dogs, ice cream, pasta, and pizza in my daily diet. I simply, and accidently, reduced the amount of food I was consuming, and I moved my body a lot more.

Let me repeat that: I simply, and accidently, reduced the amount of food I was consuming, and I moved my body a lot more.

It was simple to understand why this worked a few years later, when I started learning about nutrition and exercise. And now, as a mature man, I can easily see how this job and respect for/from Louie offered a new, positive way for me to meet my insatiable need for certainty and significance in my life—a much more positive way than chasing brain freezes! But I hadn't changed any of my personal habits yet. I was still inexperienced with myself and my own emotional needs and choices. When I ate, I still ate junk food. I just got a lot less than I was used to. And I still didn't know how to, or want to, be motivated to exercise. Still, after realizing what I had just done, I really felt as if it was a new day for me. I started to dream again about what it would be like to be skinny. I started to ask myself if I ever would be skinny. Could I do it? How would I do it? Would that mean that I could get a good girlfriend? Maybe get married and have a family? Could I get a good job? Maybe I could be a cop? Or maybe I could go in the military and fight for my country the way Louie did, the way my dad did?

Whatever it meant, this was the point of acknowledgment in my story—the point where I started to take control, the point where I started to assume a high degree of personal accountability, the point where I changed my definition of "what's normal for Doug." My choice to follow *Dad Rule #3* and be a security guard had huge consequences. It changed my life; my mind; and my future. It was the point where I started to wonder what was possible. What was I really capable of if I applied myself to something? What would it mean to have hope, to dream again, and to beat my obesity demon? What would it mean to be somebody?

Honestly speaking, I was still lost without a program and without anybody to guide me. I didn't know how to harness what I had done during the Horror Nights, but I was very sure that I didn't want to regain any fat. It was confusing. I didn't have any guidance. No doctors, trainers, pills, TV shows, the Internet, books . . . or any knowledge, really. And honestly, I was too proud at first to let myself be vulnerable to other people about it. I wanted people to think that I was in control.

After several days of reckoning, I got extremely pissed off. I was scared of gaining my weight back, and I made a firm decision. I chose to fight back. I told myself that I was done. I was done with being a junior supervisor with great cleavage; I was done being an oxymoron; I was done with being a super fat guy. I was sick and tired of being sick and tired. I was tired of analyzing everything, and my mind was exhausted. I desperately wanted to change, and I finally decided that I needed to change. I realized that I needed to take control of my life and of myself—and stop letting things happen to me. I needed to grow up, man up, figure it out, and stop being passive in life. Looking back, I was much better and more valuable than what I led myself to believe, and I needed to respect myself. I needed to respect myself (even love myself) the way Louie respected me.

How did I do this? The cold, hard truth is simple: I made a choice. That's right. I made one simple choice. I chose to no longer be scared of being fat forever and do something about it. I chose to no longer accept what I thought was my fate, my genetics, and my shame of living as a fat kid. It wasn't okay anymore to be teased by other people, to be ashamed of myself and my habits, to be hurt or feel limited. I decided to stop acting like a helpless victim—because I was not a helpless victim. I chose a full life of happiness over a depressing, limited life full of fear and anxiety. I chose to make life happen, not to let life happen to me. I decided to, at all costs, figure out my fat problem and beat it! I didn't know what or how I was going to do it; I didn't know how long it would take or what other demons I would have to face. I just knew that I had to do something about it . . . anything. I chose not to let my hopes and dreams die at the bottom of an empty ice cream carton.

For the first time in a long time, I dreamed about how I really wanted to be good at what I did, maybe even the best. I started to feel ambition. I was showing myself that I wanted something more than food. I finally got my head put on straight, as they say. I chose to follow *Dad Rule #3*, which freed my mind and helped me find a purpose. Thanks, Dad. I love you!

CHAPTER 4

TUNA BREATH

Negative self talk costs more than even the richest person can afford.
So be nice to yourself whenever possible . . . and know that it is always
possible.

—Doug Pedersen

D o you believe that pride is a deadly sin? I imagine that most people feel pride at one point in their lives and don't take the "sin" part too seriously. I had a buddy who used to be so proud of every little thing he did that he couldn't help but share it with everybody, like a peacock strutting his stuff all the time. On the other hand, I had a girlfriend who was just the opposite. She was quiet and humble, but at times her face beamed with joy while sharing facts about teeth. She was a dental student and proud to be able to pick out gingivitis and gumboils from color photos. Even my high school's motto was "pride." We were the Burbank Bulldogs, and PRIDE was painted in large white letters all over the campus, on our school T-shirts, and in the middle of our football field.

Deadly sin or not, I couldn't help but feel extremely proud after losing twenty-five fluke pounds in 1992—like the "proud parent of an honor roll student," I imagine. I didn't feel better than anyone else for doing this (not yet anyway), which is the type of pride I believe the "experts" classify as a deadly sin. I just felt good enough (proud enough) to finally take a chance at getting my childhood confidant to like me.

My childhood confidant was something I loved to hate: the weight scale that sat on my parents' bathroom floor. For me, this confidant, this mentor, this evil weight loss tool, ruled over much of my obsessive behavior, especially in the early years. I first accepted the scale's strong opinion on things in 1985, when I was eleven and just coming to grips with my super fatness. It assumed its power position the very same day I got all worked up over my hanging belly and plump man boobs. Instead of comforting me when I stood on it, the scale took on the personality of Hannibal Lecter (the mind-twisting psychiatrist) and communicated with me through the scale's digital screen (like an electronic message sign you see in Times Square). These messages registered more than a weight total too. To me, they were raw bits of emotional truths that were packed with influence. The first thing it ever said to me was, "Hey, fat boy! Did you like E.T.? Of course . . . I can tell. You look like you ate the little booger!" What kid wouldn't react to that?

Hannibal's edge did dull at times, which is why he (it) reminded me of one of my buddy's pets. My friend's family owned a dog and a cat. Spot was their black-and-white Dalmatian that lived to be one hundred dog years old. Despite becoming senile in his old age, he was the type of dog that would gladly grab you a beer out of the fridge when he was up. Friendly and affectionate, Spot never met a person he didn't like, and he never had anything bad to bark at anybody. He was a joker too. Spot often waltzed through the den with a big smirk on his face. Within seconds, his Puppy Chow farts usually followed, invading our nostrils and proving that Spotsy also believed in the universal truth of, "Whoever smelt it, dealt it." We loved him for his antics; Hannibal was nothing like this.

Their cat's name was Tiger. She was an indoor/outdoor cat that had a matching personality. Actually, I always felt that Tiger had a split personality: soft and affectionate at times, aggressive and dangerous at times—perhaps like a real tiger. Once you got to know her, Tiger was the type of cat that would snuggle up and loved to be petted. She could purr for hours while you stroked the back of her ears or the soft fur under her chin. Tiger would close her eyes and bask in the comfort, like a person getting a great Swedish massage. Within a split second, though, she would open her eyes, lift her head, and quickly bite your fingers or scratch your forearm with her razor-sharp claws as if you were a dangerous predator that she needed to attack. Tiger could only purr so long before she scratched; she could only sleep so long before she pounced; and she could only love you so long before you hated her.

Hannibal was a tiger, and I always wanted him to purr like one. So what if he had a mind-bending edge? I always figured that his sharp tongue was just a defense mechanism because he was sentenced to lying on the floor and licking people's feet all day. So what if we had longer-than-normal conversations? I was more concerned with what Hannibal thought about me, and I was sometimes scared of what he would say and ask me to do. But still, there was something in the way he talked to me—or talked down to me. I was vulnerable to it, and I always wanted his approval. At first, I just wanted him to be nice. In time, though, I wanted him to love me even when I thought there was a better chance of becoming a five-hundred-pound man with an air filter lodged in my butt crack. Somehow, Hannibal, that scale, had the ability to draw me in like the Bermuda Triangle and make me talk as if I had taken three shots of truth serum.

Perhaps it was the fact that I could be insecure in front of him as I got older. In junior or senior high school, if I whined to Hannibal, all I would risk is a few insults thrown at me across his digital screen. It was the perfect relationship for an insecure binger like me. Hannibal didn't go to my school, and we didn't know any of the same people; he wasn't in my circle of friends at all. If I opened up to him and complained about my pregnant belly or Texas toast-filled butt cheeks, which I often did, he could never blab about it to my other friends. So in the end, being vulnerable to Hannibal was as safe as talking to a priest in confessional—except that he didn't listen very well and his advice often made me feel like ass.

We had many heart-to-heart conversations, but not before Hannibal greeted me with his warmest welcome when I stepped on him: "Hello, fat boy. Well, you're still nice and blubbery to me." He thought he was a real comedian with the "nice and blubbery" routine. In my most insecure moments, I would ask him if he thought I was fat or how fat he thought I was. He wasn't a great counselor at all, but he tried to comfort me with his best one-liners.

"Hey, fat boy, you're so fat, you make Big Bird look like a rubber duck."

"Hey, fat boy, you're so fat that when you haul ass, do you have to make two trips?"

"Hey, fat boy, you're so fat that if you get a flesh-eating disease, you'll have ten years to live."

Accidentally losing twenty-five pounds as a fresh high school graduate in 1992 during the Halloween Horror Nights at the Studios was just the news I could share with Hannibal. Naturally, I ran to him to show off my smaller gut the minute Lovable Louie told me to switch out my uniforms for ones that fit. I stood in his presence and prepared for his insults.

"Hey, Hannibal, how do I look?"

"Hello, fat boy. Well, you're still nice and blubbery to me!"

"Yeah, yeah—I know. Guess what?"

"Umm, your lunch waitress gave you an estimate instead of a menu?"

"Stop it. No, I think I did something . . . something impossible."

"Did you finally do a handstand without your belly hitting your face? No, wait . . . did you lose a little weight, fat boy?"

"Can you tell—really?"

"Of course, numbnuts. I'm a scale, remember? How did you do it?"

"I got really busy at work and didn't eat, I guess."

"I got busy at work!" he mocked in a high voice.

"Seriously—do you think I can lose more?" I stood clutching my fat gut.

"Do you think you can keep forgetting to eat?"

"Maybe. Maybe this is my chance. How much do I have to lose before you're nice to me?"

"Fat boy . . . really? But you love it when I make you feel pitiful! I'll think about it, but you'd better keep forgetting to eat."

I wasn't playing with Hannibal. I did believe that this was my chance and whether he was nice to me or not, I had my eye on another love affair. I didn't tell anybody but I was falling in love with the idea of becoming a United States Marine. Maybe I was romanced by all the stuff I learned from Louie, or perhaps their recruiting campaigns were designed for young men like me. Their slogans spoke to my newly awakened ego and stoked my competitive flames in ways that nothing ever had. Can you blame me? The hairs on my neck would literally stand at attention and my skin would ripple in awe when I imagined the crisp snare drum roll playing behind phrases like "The Few. The Proud. The Marines." "We don't promise you a rose garden." "Only the best can claim the title. Do you have what it takes?" "Devil Dog!" "Shock Troop!" "Warrior!" "Leatherneck!" I was romanced; I was in love; I was horny for it.

The Marines offered the right amount of validation I needed. Becoming a badass would put me in another class. Instead of being fat, weak, and the butt of all jokes, I thought I would be lean, mean, and the cream in girls' jeans (my apologies, ladies, but that's how my arrogant young mind worked at the time). I could prove to myself and to my dad and brother that I wasn't a quitter like the one I had demonstrated on the football field. I could be strong like them too. I would be important. I could serve my country and experience true sacrifice. I could earn my freedom. I loved these ideas, and I wanted it! I wanted it more than I wanted food, and I took the next eight months proving that point to myself.

No matter what Hannibal said, I left that conversation with a new perspective. I had caught lightning in a bottle by losing twenty-five pounds, and I wasn't going to let it go. I was going to lose weight and make him be nice to me once and for all. Why? Because I was sick and tired of being super fat.

How was I, of all people, going to pull this off? I wondered. I was an impulsive binge eater after all. You would think that I would look to groups like Overeaters Anonymous, but I was too proud and hardheaded for that. Instead, I decided to follow Hannibal's advice and quit food altogether. That's right; my master plan was to quit food cold turkey. Why not? There wasn't anyone to tell me that it was a stupid idea—not that I asked anyone. Dr. Phil wasn't around to tell me that the odds of succeeding were low. What odds? I'm not sure there were obesity odds in 1992-93.

Was I really planning to be anorexic? Maybe just a little . . . or perhaps I was planning to be quasi-anorexic. In either case, I didn't label it, and I didn't feel anorexic, despite the fact that I became deathly afraid of gaining any weight back. I was more obsessed with my fat body—belly, boobs, and "Grande buttocks Canyon"—and I just wanted them to disappear. I believed that this was my only route, especially if I was ever going to make it to the Marines. So that was the master plan that I came up with.

Quitting food cold turkey was harder at first than I expected. After all, I was a binge eater. Trying to ignore my stomach's cry for food was like a young parent trying to ignore his newborn's cry for attention. The "cries" were so loud and gut twisting; I knew what my stomach wanted. In the end, fear propelled me, the "Marine dream motivated me, success emboldened me—and pride kept me ignorant to any other options.

Staying away from food was toughest the first few days and weeks. Many times when I wasn't at work, I found myself circling food like a dirty buzzard in the African desert. The minute a hunger pang would hit, I would waddle to the kitchen and rummage through the cupboards, eyeballing the Pop-Tarts, popcorn, and other foods I had stashed. Without fail and with my Pop-Tarts in the toaster, I would think about Hannibal and trash the tarts without eating them—but not before circling over to the refrigerator and gazing at the cheese slices, cherry ice cream, and chocolate bars I worked to hide from the rest of the family. I hovered over the door and drooled.

I managed to stay busy once I left the house, but the temptation to eat usually became almost unbearable on my drive home from work—mainly because our neighborhood had a most excellent array of fast-food choices. This arrangement was perfect for a practiced binge-eating teenager but torture on a newly created quasi-anorexic. There was a mile-long strip of fast-food restaurants that was like a drive-through buffet: Pioneer Chicken, McDonald's, Burger King, Wendy's, Pizza Hut, Kentucky Fried Chicken, Tommy's (home of the Original hamburger), El Rancho, Sub King, and Carl's Junior. You name it—it was there.

Before quitting food, I used to visit a drive-through and pick up lots of goodies from (m)any of my favorite restaurants. After quitting food, I would stop at a few of them just to stare at the menus, letting my mouth water before speeding away while the kid on the microphone repeated "Hello? May I take your order?" for the third time. It was torture, but I held out.

When I felt like I couldn't resist my buzzard instincts anymore, I would go see Hannibal. His rare brand of encouragement was priceless to a guy like me (a self-pitying binger) when we would have an exchange like this:

"Hello, fat boy. Well, you're still nice and blubbery to me!"

"I'm dying over here, Hannibal. I'm so hungry. How do I look?"

"Fat boy, you still make Free Willy look like a Tic Tac. Try eating those?"

He could always talk sense into me or beat me up with his insults until I felt guilty even thinking about food. I obsessively "checked in" with Hannibal so that he could brow beat the hunger pangs out of me. Sometimes I would go see him ten or fifteen times in a row before going to work just to see if he thought I *looked* skinnier. Maybe I was a little obsessed, but at least talking to Hannibal and airing my insecurities kept me out of the refrigerator. I wanted food terribly, but I was more afraid of gaining weight and just couldn't bring myself to eat.

Within a short time of quitting food, I adapted my habits accordingly. Buzzards are only attracted by dead carcasses, so throwing my food stash away made sense. I gutted the cupboards like a fish so that if I felt the impulse to scavenge, I would only find empty shelves. I changed my route home too. Instead of driving the food gauntlet, I started driving home on side streets, avoiding the drive-through menus altogether. At work, Louie stopped asking me for ice cream chats because he knew I was horny for the Marines. He was in my corner and the only one I really told (except for my brother). I simply pulled away from anybody else that might influence or put junk food in front of me. I stayed away from the Riverboat, from buddies I used to hang out with during meal times, and so forth. I just pulled away.

Quitting food cold turkey eventually became impossible. Like any vulnerable dieter, I caved when I couldn't take it anymore, thereby risking my entire plan. The first time I ate, the fear boiled my blood like volcano lava because I was sure that I had added inches back to my waistline. I had to see Hannibal. This was an emergency.

"Hello, fat boy. Well, you're still nice and blubbery to me. Why the long face?"

"I had to do it, Hannibal. I feel like I ran over a puppy, but I just had to do it."

"Aye, fat boy, what happened? Did you get a speeding ticket going through the buffet line again?" he cackled from his spot on the floor.

"I just ate, and I'm afraid I gained some weight back. Can you tell?"

"Fat boy, why do you smell like cat food?"

"I found a small can of tuna and some soda crackers. I think I gained at least a pound."

"You *are* crazy, eh. Listen, you didn't gain a pound, and you're not going to die. Stick with it and see what happens. I'll tell you if you get more *blubbery.*"

So that's what I did. When my stomach yelled and complained about being empty, I simply absorbed the pain as long as I could and waited it out. By the time I couldn't take it anymore, I prepared a meal fit for a kitten: one small can of tuna (plain), three soda crackers, and two oranges. I ate this royal feast only once a day (maybe)—usually for lunch. The rest of the time, I water boarded my stomach throughout the day, drowning it with quart-size helpings of diet iced tea from my favorite Carl's Junior mug.

I kept this routine as if it were my job, and the "tuna experiment" became surprisingly easy after the first month. Looking back, fear propelled me, the Marine dream motivated me, success emboldened me—and my pride kept me ignorant to any other options. Who knew that I scared myself into not eating? Who knew that I was deathly afraid of gaining any weight back and anxious about missing my window with the Marine Corps? Perhaps like a woman whose biological clock is ticking, I was ripe at nineteen and felt my "Marine clock" ticking. It was urgent. If I didn't sign a contract soon, I would be too old, as most guys sign up while still in high school. Tuna and oranges was my staple and quasi-anorexia became my new normal.

I shed another fifty pounds by quitting food cold turkey, but regular exercise really kicked my weight loss into overdrive. Hannibal, of all "people," motivated me to start by giving me a speech that was much less inspiring and instructive than Richard Simmons':

"Hello, fat boy. Well, you're still nice and blubbery to me! You look thinner, but if you ran away, they would still have to use two sides of the milk carton for your picture."

That day, I bought a pair of running shoes, and like Forrest Gump, I started to run. I ran up hills, I ran down streets, I ran down trails, and I ran on tracks. I just ran. Walking at work was the only exercise I had gotten in years, so I started out on the track at my old high school. Of course, it was only hard at first.

Quitting food cold turkey got easier as time went on. Fear propelled me, the Marine dream motivated me, success emboldened me—and pride kept me ignorant to any other options. It became my routine, and eating a can of tuna once a day was my new normal. Ironically, I was a fat guy who had more than acid reflux swirling up from his belly. I found that I had a lot of discipline hidden in there somewhere for a long time. Somehow, I had sacrifice and the iron willpower of a stubborn jackass mule—a lot of it. Funny thing: I was actually "born to starve." Once I got into it, it was easy; it was my *new* binge. These characteristics were going to serve me very well in the Marines, I arrogantly thought: *Survival, adapt and overcome, do more with less.* I was made for it, but how would I have ever known unless I stopped eating Riverboat hot dogs out of the trash can and tried to eat less?

The truth is I gave myself a super-sized portion of what some would call "tough love." In reality, though, I served myself more enormous helpings of negative self-talk that literally dismissed the desire to eat out of my body. Anyway, lucky for me, and without realizing it at the time, fat is actually a rich energy source. There are nine calories (or units of energy the body can use) in one gram of fat. Doing nothing else, the human body can burn nine calories in every 150 breaths (within eighteen to twenty minutes). It's not ideal, but I basically created a huge calorie deficit. By adding some minor activity at work and moving around throughout the day I was able to keep functioning "normally" without eating hardly anything. Looking back, it's hard to say that I starved myself. I had stored fat for ten years—way longer than a hibernating bear does before he goes down for the winter—and I had a lot of energy (fat) to burn up.

Most people were struck by my weight loss but couldn't tell that I was starving, that I was rejecting food altogether. I hid that too. A buddy at work asked if I was sick; my parents just thought that I was eating a lot of tuna; and most people didn't say anything. Maybe they were stunned by my rapid transformation. My body had no choice. I was probably getting less than five hundred calories per day, when I maybe could've consumed three times that and still lost weight. The fat melted off my bones like hot candle wax rolling off its wick, which made me crave hunger more and more.

"Skinny Doug" surprised Hannibal too. Eight months in to my tuna experiment, it was time to ask him if he was ready to be nice to me forever. Hannibal was lying in his usual spot on the floor. I stepped on him to check my weight and admire my new body, but Hannibal scolded me instead.

"Be nice to you? No way! Have you looked in the mirror lately, jellyfish?"

"Yeah . . . I guess?"

"Did you notice that you're a stick figure with loose-hanging skin? Don't you get it? I'll never be nice to weak turds like you!"

Goddammit! As much as I hated him right then, I let Hannibal be right again. He always was. The fact is that I had lost 125 pounds in eight months—in the blink of an eye, really. Somehow, I had finally waved a magic wand to make my pregnant belly, beautiful set of boobs, and giant ass cheeks vanish while keeping my lanky six-foot frame. I was born to be skinny, but not that skinny. I looked like the frail AIDs-stricken lawyer that Tom Hanks played in *Philadelphia*. I had clearly gone too far. I was a bag of bones and loose skin.

Quitting food cold turkey got easier as time went on. Fear propelled me, the Marine dream motivated me, success emboldened me, and pride kept me ignorant to any other options.

Life and Hannibal—what *teases* sometimes!

CHAPTER 5

RUN, FORREST, RUN!

Now you wouldn't believe me if I told you, but I could run like the wind blows. From that day on, if I was ever going somewhere, I was running!

—*Forrest Gump*

My mom, God bless her, is a real angel. I don't know about yours, but mine has delicately and quietly watched over me all my life. Through thick and thin, ups and downs, happy and sad, fat and thin, Mom was the one who always offered a ray of light and a beaming smile. To say that she's the best mother in the world might be an understatement. The truth is, I'm not really sure where or who I would be today if she wasn't the one who raised me. Some things are certain, though: I would probably be less optimistic, less understanding, and much less patient. Perhaps I'd spend my days peering out of a garbage can on a corner somewhere telling people to scram, to go away and leave me alone.

Her name is Anne—or just plain "Ma" to me—and she would likely remind you of a sweet farm girl from the Great Plains of Nebraska. As the only female in our house, it's safe to say that she kept my dad, brother, and me from reverting into cavemen that spoke in grunts, traded scratching techniques, and cooked everything over an open flame. There's no doubt that Ma classed the place up a lot! She was the keeper of the nest, and she made sure that we ate more than what could be cooked on a barbecue. For me, she was safe: Ma let me suck my fingers, play with a *silky* (one of her old slips that felt like silk), and throw pot holders around the kitchen—things my dad and older brother probably just didn't get. More importantly, Ma nurtured us and always encouraged us to think for ourselves. Instead of commanding Ben and me to do things, Ma gently influenced us with questions: "What if you try it this way, son?" and "How do you like that?" and "How about putting it this way?" and "What if this . . . ?" and "What if that . . . ?" and "Do you need to go wet-wet?"

Ma didn't seem to require a lot of unnecessary structure or have strict rules around the house. Dad was the keeper of the rules (remember *Dad Rules*). He was the disciplinarian, the *heavy*. Ma was the one who showed us how to make animal shapes out of Play-Doh—and when she turned her back, we'd make boogers and such. Ma gave us crayons and construction paper to draw on at the kitchen table. I drew stick figures and Mr. Potato Head characters with goofy smiles and missing teeth. She sent us outside a lot to ride our skateboards and bikes or just climb trees. Ma also gave us little jobs like clearing the table and washing the dishes, even as very little guys, until my brother Ben and I learned to be independent, acting like little-big people even at ages three, four, and five.

I always figured that *that's* how farm people did it. Ma was one of eight brothers and sisters; Dad was one of ten. My friends had different experiences with their parents, like divorce and adultery, but that never mattered much to me. Maybe that's why I never really noticed that we didn't have a lot of extra money around. My parents didn't even have a television in the house until I was eight or nine. Instead, Ma took time in the evenings to sit with us and read books. She read us many novels, but our favorite was *The Chronicles of Narnia*. She loved reading us those stories, and we loved listening to her. On any given night, my dad might be working one of his two or three jobs, whereas my mom would take her spot in the middle of couch. "Okay, boys, are you ready to hear the next adventure?" Without any more coaxing, Ben and I eagerly stopped whatever foolishness we were up to and raced to the couch to take our places on either side of her. Ma started the story from the page she left off the night before as we laid our heads on her lap, listening as her soft inflections took over the room and the wild stories of Edmund, Lucy, Peter, and Aslan took over our active imaginations.

Ma never gave up her caretaker role as we got older either. I remember one time when I was seven years old. I complained to my dad about a toothache, and he told me to suck on an aspirin, so I did. (I told you: cavemen!) None of us knew any better back then, except for Ma. The aspirin tasted like bitter chalk that had been aged in a rhino's ass for decades, but I kept it in my mouth nonetheless. I meandered around the house, forgetting all about my tooth but wondering now if my tongue would fall out, and finally Ma intervened. She must have noticed my face start to cave in, and when she discovered an aspirin halfway dissolved between my cheek and gum, she quickly had me spit it out. What a relief! She got me to the dentist . . . but not before explaining to my dad how aspirin worked.

Now don't get me wrong. I'm not a mama's boy, and my mother was no slouch. But the fact is Ma was too sweet to discipline us. I figure she just couldn't bring herself to raise her hands in a forceful way against her little guys—even when we deserved it! But that didn't mean that she was a weak pushover. Remember *Dad Rule #1: Don't piss off your mother?* Well, let's just say that the quickest way to get spanked in our house was to break that rule—and with Dad's intimidating size, you didn't want to be on his bad side. Dad kept a spanking stick in the closet that looked more like a Louisville Slugger to a kid like me. It was the peacemaker and Ma's nuclear option. Five or six swift swats to the ass made you quickly regret whatever smart-ass remark you said or whatever thing you did. I knew that the swats were on their way every time I heard her say, "Wait until your father gets home!" The second time I heard her say that (and every time after that), my throat dropped to the pit of my stomach as my sphincter clinched shut.

Anyway, like an angel, Ma was more interested in guiding us than spanking us. She saw this as her job, and it's no wonder she continued to care as I got into my teenage years. I always thought that it must have been hard for her at times as she watched me gain weight and become obese. I'm sure it even broke her heart from time to time, not really knowing how to help me. But I don't think she could have. Ma didn't see me as a binge eater, and I rarely complained to her about being fat. Ma was safe; she never changed the way she looked at me. She never judged me as I gained weight or nagged me for lacking direction and ambition. She just kept listening, encouraging, and nurturing. She always suggested and always loved—always.

It was only natural that Ma paid casual attention to my choices after I graduated high school. Not that I noticed much, but I suppose I looked aloof and without direction. Sure, my wheels were always grinding, and my silent dreams of being a Marine were always on my mind. But Ma was left completely in the dark, which must have made my nurturing and forever present guardian angel a little antsy.

I remember her divine intervention as if it were yesterday. I had no idea that it was coming, as I wasn't expecting her to nudge me down a certain life path—but she did. It was during the holiday season of 1992—my senior year in high school and the year prior to my "tuna experiment" and significant weight loss. Without a lot of drama, we had a conversation about my future. Actually, one day before work, I found her sitting in the kitchen. I was walking through to get a snack, and she invited me to sit down at the breakfast nook with her. I sat down on the green vinyl bench seat. The lamp hung over us and illuminated a small packet of papers that were neatly stacked in front of her. Those papers were carefully laid down on the table like an unsuspecting bear trap, and somehow my quick trip for Pop-Tarts turned into a completed application to Los Angeles Valley College.

"You haven't talked about the SATs in a while, Doug. Have you thought more about going to college?"

"Kind of . . . ," I mumbled back, still not getting what was going on.

The truth is that I *had* thought a lot about going to college during my senior year. Why not? My counselor forced me to take the advanced placement (college-level) courses, and I did well in them. Most if not all of those kids were headed to UCLA or UC San Diego, so why not me? I even took the SATs and made my parents take a campus tour of USC before I applied there. But after I received my rejection letter later in the year, I quickly put college out of my mind. They didn't want me, and I didn't want them. I never expressed any of that to my mother (to either of my parents, really). Instead, I went along with her program, opting not to piss her off (*Dad Rule #1*, I guess.) Mom glanced at the stack of papers and slowly revealed the brochure to Valley. "It's on the way to work, Doug," she said. "Maybe you can find something you're interested in there?"

I nodded my head as she slowly walked me through the application. In fact, I'm pretty sure she filled it in too. It didn't take long. There's a longer application process to work at McDonald's than there is to be a student at Valley College. But we filled it out anyway. I sat there in the nook and answered every question as if I were actually interested in going, when the truth was that I really didn't think I could be bothered with more classroom time after I left high school. Still, Ma had no idea where my mind was at. How could she? I'd never told her that I thought Valley College was for suckers.

However motivated I appeared to my mother at that time, the aloof slacker in me quickly reappeared when I went to the campus bookstore the following fall season in preparation for the 1993 spring semester. I couldn't have been less interested in being there, still fat, wandering the aisles and wondering what the return policy was. My required book list had twelve entries minimum, and I quit looking after only finding three of them. *I'll just copy off someone else*, I thought. *It's only Valley.*

My interest in being great at community college dropped even more when I looked around at the other students. I remember standing in line at the registration office waiting to pay my tuition. The line was at least fifty kids deep, and everyone was much more excited than I to be there. Of course, I stood next to a pack of giggling girls who couldn't wait for classes to start. They were excited about Valley—who their teachers were, which friends they shared classes with, and which benches to eat lunch at in the quad. On the other side, I saw nerds with full book bags. Apparently, they could navigate the bookstore shelving system and find all their required reading. There were preppies, jocks, cool kids, and nerdy kids, but I didn't see anyone like me.

I didn't see anyone who didn't want to be there. I didn't see anyone who had other ambitions or who wanted to be a Marine (that dream was awakened in me by this time). All I could see was Van Nuys—the city next to Burbank where Valley College was, the same town that Rodney King and the Las Angeles Police Department made famous the year before. I saw it as a dark place, full of nothing creative or fun, void of opportunity, the place where kids with no futures or money ended up. This Valley of losers was not for me and I judged it/them harshly.

Nothing changed when I met my first teacher. His name was Mr. Cook, and he taught English literature—another subject I cared absolutely nothing about. He was a nice enough guy, I suppose, but he was about as inspiring as a swift kick to the groin. Cook stood five feet four inches if he stood a foot. His shiny bald head and chubby face sat atop his rotund body. Cook always looked happy, but that's because his cheeks were puffy, giving him a natural grin even when his face was at rest. The same puffy cheeks made his eyes squint even when they were wide open. He wore lots of brown slacks, cream dress shirts, and a brown plaid jacket every day—like it was his uniform. Cook walked slowly and talked slowly, which made it easy to think of him as a turtle.

Cook's low monotone voice was soothing and encouraged me to sleep. His quotes from Hamlet sounded like the motion of the ocean to my ears, and it was easy not to retain his words. The only words I remember Cook saying were, "Does that register?" It was like his catchphrase. "Does that register?" usually followed a torturously long, slow, and impossible-to-follow explanation of the finer plot points of *Oedipus Rex.* As such, "Does that register?" usually signaled me to wipe the drool that strung from my mouth to the desktop and shuffle out the door with the other drones . . . er, kids.

The only thing that truly registered about Cook's class was how he could make me daydream. Many times in those instances, I let my mind wander until I started thinking about running. Yep, me, the lazy fat kid, would often daydream about running. My "tuna experiment" was well underway, by mid-semester, and I used to wonder how far the Marines would make me run, if I would ever make it, and if I would ever be good at it. I wondered how many laps around the classroom equaled a mile, and I wondered how far I would have to run to get away from Cook and people like him. I wondered about running, and I visualized taking step after step after step. Running was the key to everything. Running would make me lose my fat faster and allow me to stop starving myself. Running would get me recruited by the Marines. Running would get me out of the Valley of losers and out of my security guard job. Running became my new obsession, and I sure became a running fool.

It didn't take long before Cook's class became an afterthought, like the rest of Valley College, and I started ditching classes again. Only instead of ditching to listen to Howard Stern, I ditched to go run and work on my distance and speed. It took a little time for me to muster the courage to run during the day, so I started running at night in the dark so that no one, including me, could see my embarrassment. Of course, it was hard, and it seemed damn impossible at first because instead of possessing a smooth, powerful stride like a puma, my running stride still looked like a giant baby hopping down the road. But at least I was moving.

Within a few weeks, I moved my running to the track at my old high school. I worked up to the point where I could jog a lap and walk a lap . . . jog a lap and walk a lap. I stayed consistent and never missed a workout; I just wanted it so bad. It was easy to skip class, skips meals, skip the opportunity to learn anything, or skip out on making new friends. I didn't care about anything except missing a running workout—it just didn't happen. I ran so much that it became an obsession. I dropped the rest of my weight like a hot rock and found my running stride.

I was a running fool. I ran with my shirt off. I ran in the middle of the day. I ran in the open. I ran far; I ran free. I wanted everyone to see me. I timed myself and I got increasingly faster the minute I started keeping track. I pushed myself as I never had—as I never knew I could do—to the point where I was running a mile and a half in just over eight minutes, faster than everyone else in my recruiting class. Who would've thought that running was my hidden talent? Some get magic, some get acting, and some get writing skills; I got a runner's body that was hidden by years of binge eating and insecurity. No one, including me, could've seen that one coming. When I wasn't running, it was difficult to think about school at all. My entire focus was centered on becoming a Marine and even when I was at work, I thought about and looked for opportunities to run. Boy, I sure was a running fool.

One day during that first semester at Valley, Louie asked me if I wanted to do a special assignment. As it turns out, Bob Hope was coming to the lot to watch *Jurassic Park* with his wife. Bob was apparently a close friend of the CEO's, and Louie wanted me to be part of the escort team. It would just be Louie and me, so of course I agreed. "Remember, he's just another old guy going to watch a dinosaur flick with his wife. Don't say anything stupid; leave the wisecracks to the real comedian. Got it?" Louie politely suggested.

Louie didn't have to worry; I wasn't going to say anything at all. My job wasn't to entertain Bob. In his briefing, Louie told me that our biggest risk was from someone seeing Bob Hope as an opportunity to get a free souvenir. He went on to explain that most people would recognize him and want an autograph or something, but there was likely a teenager or some type of grifter that may want to take the opportunity to swipe a piece of property from the Hollywood star. I figured that Louie asked me along in case I needed to chase someone down. Of course, I turned the assignment into a running assignment.

The movie day finally came. It was warm outside, and the bright sun cooked the blacktop that Louie and I were positioned on in front of the theater as we waited to for the car to arrive. We must have stood there waiting for an hour, and all I could think about was running. I was on alert, looking for would-be autograph seekers, looky-loos, and souvenir stealers. The black limousine approached from the bottom of the hill. Louie waved the driver in, and without a lot of buildup, the back door casually opened and a sharply dressed elderly gentleman in a beige leisure suit and pure white Panama hat slowly exited the car. It was Bob Hope—live and in color. His trademark jaw line and grin led the way, and I couldn't help but think that he must have been the most famous person I ever saw. People young and old recognized him. He was loved by all, and it created quite a stir when folks caught a glimpse of the aging performer.

Bob didn't speak much, but his voice still carried the same crisp and high pitches it had as a young man. It was unmistakable. "Come, Dolores. It's this way."

Louie approached the star with care and said, "Mr. Hope. My name is Lou Sale. This is my partner, Doug Pedersen. Mr. Wasserman sent us. We'll be taking care of you today. Right this way, sir." He motioned with his now ice cream—free hand.

Mr. Hope slowly turned to Dolores and asked, "Are you *gettin'* all that?"

Louie winked in my general direction. *Another old guy coming to watch a dinosaur flick with his wife,* I thought as we led them to their private row inside the theater.

With Louie positioned on one side and me on the other, the couple was fairly isolated. I could tell that Louie was on full cop alert. He must've done plenty of private security details to earn extra money when he was a young cop. Even in the dark, I could feel his eyes scanning rows, scanning the Hopes', scanning me. Every few minutes I would look over to see what he was doing, only to catch Bob loudly whispering, "Are you *gettin'* all that?"

I tried taking my cues from Louie, but I still couldn't help myself from thinking about running. I remember focusing on Bob's white Panama hat, figuring that if anything, that's the item that a souvenir stealer would go for. So I imagined what I would do if someone reached up from behind my left shoulder and plucked the white hat clean off of Bob Hope's head. I would jump up and chase the gypsy down and tackle him before he made it to the popcorn stand—maybe even before the slushy stand. You would think I would be immersed in the movie, the beautiful scenery, the action of the dinosaurs, the superior acting of Jeff Goldbloom—something . . . anything. All I could think about was taking action and chasing someone to recover Bob Hope's white Panama hat.

We ate at Gladstones seafood restaurant after the movie. Bob and Dolores sat in a booth next to ours. Bob took his hat off and set it on the counter that shaped his booth. I focused on it like a well-trained bird dog. He couldn't have cared less about the hat, however, as he continued to ask Dolores, "Did you get all that?" Bob didn't need to care about his hat, because I did. It was now off his head and unsecured, and I thought for sure that someone might choose to boost it. So I kept one leg in the aisle in case I needed to dart out and chase someone.

Louie looked at me strangely and said, "You okay over there? Go ahead and hit the men's if you need to; Bob isn't going anywhere for a while." Of course, I didn't need to pee, and nothing ever happened.

After dinner, Bob wanted to walk down the Universal CityWalk. I was so amped. This was the first time that the public at large would truly have access to him during his entire visit. My adrenaline pumped, and I thought for sure that a gang of gypsies would strike at any minute. That white hat stayed in my view the entire time. I walked on my toes in order to avoid getting caught flat-footed. There was no way that Panama hat was going anywhere except back on top of Bob Hope's head and into the black limousine it had arrived in. Of course, Bob's stroll down the walk was uneventful. The people smiled as they passed by and followed closely, clearly just wanting to be near him in case he said something funny.

What can I say? I just felt like running—or in this case, chasing. Somehow, Bob's white Panama hat triggered something in me. I hadn't chased anything in years, except for a good food coma. I couldn't see the irony then, but the fact is that even in high school, I had decided that I would never run, not even if I was going to get my ass kicked. My thought process was this: *Even if I'm going to get my ass kicked, at least it will be with lungs full of air!* Now I was daydreaming about chasing gypsy women down the streets of LA.

Looking back, I rather surprised myself because I had never reacted like that before, and I looked for more opportunities to take action at work. I found myself doing more and more running too. When Vince Neil from Mötley Crüe and his entourage got into a backstage brawl at the amphitheater, I was the first one there because I ran when I heard the call go out over the radio. I did the same thing when Michael Jackson made a surprise appearance at the Studio Store. It was supposed to be Michael J. Fox—that's the word we got—but when it turned out to be Michael Jackson, I had to run and create a barricade before the King of Pop was literally trampled by the frenzy of tourists that hadn't expected to see him that day. And I found myself running after shoplifters—tackled one guy in the grass as if I were Brian Urlacker himself.

Who had I become? Valley College was a serious afterthought behind all this action, with all this running to do. Somewhere under one hundred pounds of lazy couch potato, I had uncovered a jackrabbit that yearned to spring into action at the drop of a white Panama hat. My hidden talent, indeed. I sure was a running fool. Funny thing: I couldn't even see the rapid changes to my personality that came along with the rapid physical changes to my body.

In running so fast and so often, I didn't see that I was also running away from my old self and from who I truly was. In essence, I did a mad dash away from the obese kid, away from the guy who shied away from competition and confrontation, who was quick to act cool and aloof on the outside while burning in pain on the inside. All that starving and sacrifice. All that running at night and during the day. All that daydreaming and avoiding Mr. Cook and Valley College like the plague. I was not running to lose weight. I was running to qualify for the Marines. I was running away from my past. I was running into someone who was unrecognizable, to someone new—someone I didn't know, couldn't have foreseen, or couldn't control. In all that running, I was losing more than my fatty shell. I was also losing the identity that came along with it. I couldn't have cared less about Valley College, Mr. Cook, or anyone there. I was becoming holier than thou, unrecognizable . . . literally and figuratively.

A few weeks after the Hopes' visit, I went to breakfast with my parents. My parents set aside Saturday mornings to eat breakfast together and catch up on the week's events. This Saturday was a special one. It was late May, and my inaugural semester at Valley College was going nowhere fast. My older brother, Ben, was home from his two-year stint in the Army. My parents loved Ben very much, and even though they loved and treated us equally, Ben was special because he was the oldest. He was special because he was first. He was in charge first. He was in trouble first. He was celebrated first. It all made sense to me because he was also out of the womb first.

But something significant happened that day that I will never, ever forget. It truly branded my transformation and triggered a runner's response that took me almost fifteen years to understand and reverse. As we finished our breakfast, I saw one of my high school teachers in the distance, sitting at another booth. I recognized him immediately. It was Coach Kent—the tall, thin guy with brown curly hair; I remembered him from high school. Kent always wore a ball cap and shorts. To me, he looked like Tom Selleck without the mustache. It's not as if a long time had passed, but Kent was familiar to me because I had taken his health classes, his volleyball classes, and I was his teacher's assistant for a whole school year. I had been around the guy consistently for two or three years straight, and now here he was in this restaurant. Strangers we were not.

Ben knew him well, too. Ben was one of Kent's teacher's assistants, and Ben had played junior varsity football when Kent was a coach. It had been almost one year since I graduated high school and since I had last seen Kent. Ben hadn't seen him for two years. But we had spent so much time around him, like many Burbank High School kids, and he was like the uncle who lived across town. I nudged Ben with a free elbow and pointed toward Kent's booth. "Check out Magnum. Let's go say hi."

While my dad paid the check, my brother and I excused ourselves from the table and walked up to Kent. He and Ben greeted each other immediately, with big smiles, a hard handshake, and even a bear hug—like long-lost relatives or something. I didn't think too much of it at first, but Kent and I didn't greet each other. Because Ben was fresh back from the Army, there was a lot for those two to catch up on. I figured that after talking to Ben, Kent would hug me next. When Kent asked about the Army, Ben told him about being a medic and driving an ambulance in and out of the infamous Fort Leavenworth Federal Prison.

Just as my mind started to drift from being ignored, it hit me like a ton of bricks: Kent didn't recognize me. He didn't recognize me as Ben's brother; he didn't recognize me as "Doug," the fat kid with long blond hair who used to dog his runs in PE and ditch his health classes. As Ben yammered on about the prison, I got a little excited; it was as if I were wearing a great disguise, and the implications were huge. As I stayed in my own head, my daydreaming was interrupted when Ben said, "Hey, Coach, what do you think of Doug's new look?"

Kent looked me up and down, his eyebrows crossed and his nose scrunched in confusion. He looked at me as Bob Hope had looked at *Jurassic Park*, and he said after a long pause, "Wow! Doug? I didn't recognize you without the hair, black T-shirt, and jeans."

Looking back, I shouldn't have been so surprised that he didn't recognize me. I did look remarkably different since leaving his classrooms almost nine months before. Instead of the size fifty blue jeans I wore on even the hottest days to hide my tree trunk-shaped legs, I now wore a pair of surfboard shorts with a thirty-inch waist. Instead of the black double XL T-shirts that I used to wear in any weather to slim my love handles and hide my belly, I now wore a tight OP T-shirt tucked into my waistband. Instead of the long blond hair that I let grow in front of my face to hide my sadness, I now wore a closely cropped buzz cut that was just a few millimeters longer than what the Marines would do to it once they got me in the chair.

"Yeah," I mumbled. "I've been trying to lose a few pounds."

Kent shook his head as if doing a double take, trying to uncross his eyes, I suppose, before he quickly held out his arms and hugged me while saying, "Are you sick or something? You know even Magic Johnson caught the AIDS."

Caught the AIDS? Caught the AIDS! Well, Kent had a point, and it was hard to ignore when I really let myself think about it. The loose skin around my stomach was hard to ignore, but my puny shoulders, skinny neck, and girly-man arms were toughest to hide. I went from looking like the Stay Puft Marshmallow Man to looking like every stick figure I drew as a kid. It was still better than being fat, I thought; still, I couldn't shake the impact of that moment as I really started thinking about how Kent had seen me as a stranger at first. I was unrecognizable to him. The even weirder part was that I didn't say anything at first. I didn't tell him who I was. Instead, I let him think that I was someone else, and I didn't react at all until Ben tipped him off.

Kent made me finally see my own physical transition. It was so huge and so drastic; people that knew me didn't even recognize me. I could get away with a new identity. Like a thief on the lam, I could sneak forward through life and become someone else altogether. I could change; I did change. I was different from before—more than just lighter. I saw myself in the same way when I looked in the mirror, but no one else did, and people that I met from that point forward didn't know and couldn't see my not-so-distant past that I was so ashamed of. I could be whoever I wanted to be. People, like Kent, would judge me differently now. The fat weak-minded kid was dead and unrecognizable. He had simply dropped off the face of the earth, never to be seen again. This was a green light moment, and that kid ran far, far away.

From that point on, I committed to never letting people know the truth about my obesity. I didn't tell stories to anyone, and all my childhood pictures were buried. I let my parents know over the years that I didn't want them to be seen by anyone. That guy literally disappeared; he was a mystery, a figment of everyone's imagination, especially mine, so I committed to making sure that people would see me differently from that day forth.

I showed up to class at Valley the following Monday feeling empowered, reinvigorated, and perhaps even awake. To Cook's surprise, I sat in the front row, as I was actually going to pay attention. He couldn't see my intentions, and not even I knew what I was doing there. I had already made up my mind, but I suppose I wanted him to see me one last time.

"Glad you could make it, Doug. We're taking our tests at the end of the week. I hope you're prepared. Does that register?"

I smirked and nodded my head. Cook started the lecture, and I started to daydream. Visions of running flashed through my mind. I imagined all the steps I had taken to lose my weight; I thought about the running displays I had put on for the various recruiters in town; I wondered how much running I would have to do in boot camp; I thought about running though jungles, rivers, and down beaches. I thought about Kent, and it finally registered. I was done with Valley College before I had even started.

I stuffed my pen in my pocket and closed my notebook that was full of empty scribbles, and I walked out of Cook's class for good. I didn't care if they considered me a dropout; I didn't care if they failed me. I just didn't care anymore about the Valley of losers. So I got in my car and sped away from the mental dungeon. I never looked back at Valley College. I never told a teacher, I never told a counselor, I never consulted my parents, I never opened my mail from them, and I never cared enough to care about what quitting college meant to me in the short or long run.

When I got home, I called my recruiter on the phone. I was ready, and I had decided during Cook's class that I was going to do it. It finally registered. It was time for me to sign a contract with the Marines. I had enough physical strength. I was running like the wind. I was doing sit-ups on my parents' den floor. I was doing chin-ups on my mom's clothesline in the backyard every chance I got. I was beginning to dislike people like Cook and show little patience for things that weren't going to help me get to the Marines. My competitive drive was stoked; I was ready physically, and now I was ready mentally. The Marines would never see me as an obese kid. It had registered, and now was the time.

My parents both cried when I told them. I thought that Dad would be pissed that I dropped out of college, but in his own tender, loving way, he cried and told me, "Your mom and I would be devastated if you or Ben ever came home in a body bag. We just love you so much, Doug. The Marines are lucky to have you . . ." Dad always had a sneaking suspicion that I was thinking about the Marines, but I never discussed it with him, even when I probably should have.

Mom, on the other hand, was completely taken aback by the news. She had no idea that I had been ditching classes and visiting recruiters on my own time. How could she? Since that moment in the breakfast nook, I'd kept up the appearance that things were fine and classes were going well. I suppose at times she didn't understand me, but she was extremely proud nonetheless. To this day, she was sure that Ben was meant for the military and I was not. I was more of a dreamer and someone without structure, I suppose.

In the end, all that running allowed me to run away from my past while running into the future. In the months that followed, I trained my body more and waited for my ship date. I started eating more—chicken with rice and vegetables became my new normal—and I gained twenty healthy much-needed pounds. I finally looked strong and healthy, and I was on my way.

Ma watched me run after that too, and of all the people in the world, she's one of the ones who never stopped recognizing me. She and Dad filmed my runs around Elysian Park and Dodger Stadium, playing the sound track to *Rocky III* ("Eye of the Tiger") in the background. I felt their pride. Mom went to the track with me and watched as I did sprints and pull-ups. She did the cool-down walking laps with me and listened as I sung her the Marines' Hymn. She listened to me recite the General Orders I had been memorizing when no one was looking, and she watched as my passion finally grew (or ran) toward something. Ma never stopped encouraging me. She was never judging and was always loving me—always. Thanks, Ma. I love you!

I ran to the Marines and away from my past. It was a hidden talent that I couldn't have anticipated, controlled, or changed. I'd wanted to be someone different my entire life, and now I believed that I was. My talent became running, and who would ever have guessed that the fat kid could run so fast and so far? In all that insatiable running, I was still unconsciously trying to meet my needs for significance while being shaped by something more powerful that I didn't understand. I was preparing for an adventure of a lifetime and sprinting in all directions. I had become a silent competitor—rigid, disciplined, and judgmental. Little did I know that I was still chasing Panama hats and running away from the guy that everyone knew and loved. Boy, I sure became a running fool!

CHAPTER 6

RUNNING WITH THE DEVIL

Arrogance and rudeness are training wheels on the bicycle of life, for weak people who cannot keep their balance without them.
—Laura Teresa Marquez

Many of us have seen *The Matrix* and likely remember the red and blue pills. They make their appearance early in the movie and represent a crossroad moment to the main character, Neo, played by Keanu Reeves. The pills represent deceit and truth, and the scene makes one feel the tension as Morpheus tempts Neo's fate through the length of the movie.

The scene starts with Neo entering a dimly lit room. Across the floor is a tall dark-skinned man with dapper clothes and a long duster overcoat. Calling himself Morpheus, the man says to Neo, "I imagine that right now you're feeling a bit like Alice . . . tumbling down the rabbit hole. I can see it in your eyes. You have the look of a man who accepts what he sees because he's expecting to wake up. Ironically, this is not far from the truth."

Neo *is* there to "wake up." He wants to learn the truth about the "matrix"—the computer program that has enslaved all human minds. It's then when Morpheus stretches out his hand toward Neo as he sits in the chair. Two pills are revealed in his large palm: one blue pill and one red pill.

"After this, there is no turning back," Morpheus proclaims. "You take the blue pill. The story ends. You wake up in your bed and believe . . .

whatever you want to believe. You take the red pill. You stay in Wonderland and I show you how deep the rabbit hole goes. Remember, all I'm offering is the truth. Nothing more."

Neo glances around the room at the other characters before locking eyes with Morpheus. He quickly snatches the blue pill, and the movie ends promptly. *Just kidding!* As we all know, Neo, overcome with curiosity, eagerly swallows the red pill (the truth) and gives birth to three more Hollywood blockbusters.

I'm guessing that most of us have not been offered blue pills by tall dudes named Morpheus, unless you watch a lot of late night infomercials or you're a guy who is looking to "enhance that special part of the male body." But most of us have had moments of choice, moments of conflict, just like Neo, where learning the truth about something could seriously upset the apple cart. These are crossroads, moments of growth, inflection points, or just plain events that life throws at us to guide us down certain paths. However you think of it, this was how I felt after completing Marine Combat Training (MCT)—only instead of a blue and red pill, I got Sergeant Green and Sergeant Sanchez.

For those who don't know, Marine Combat Training is exactly what it sounds like. It's the phase of training that takes place after boot camp; every Marine is required to complete it. MCT is all about weapons, field training, battle tactics, rifle platoon movements, squad movements, and bowel movements in the dirt. Only men were in this training with me— and even though we thought that boot camp was an accomplishment, thirty days of MCT changed our lives. MCT was simply about fighting.

I remember it as if it were yesterday, although it was 1994. I had just turned nineteen years old. One year before that, I was a simple security guard at Universal Studios starving on a crazy tuna and cracker diet while playing an emotional version of Russian roulette (*Am I fat . . . Am I not fat*) with my parents' bathroom scale (remember Hannibal?).

But MCT stood out in my mind compared to the first three months of my Marine Corps career (boot camp). Instead of training in an urban facility next to the San Diego airport, complete with spotless barracks and giant concrete parade decks, MCT was held at Camp Pendleton, California. Pendleton sat on the coast between Los Angeles and San Diego. Everything was green or brown, and there was hardly any flat ground. The base was organized into smaller camps that were situated miles apart from each other—separated by training areas, obstacles courses, rifle ranges, and about thirty thousand jarheads. The Southern California sunshine encouraged birds, deer, and snakes to occupy the hills, but oftentimes I could see them get chased off by a burst of machine gun fire in the distance or by a low-flying helicopter.

The ground at Camp Pendleton felt like cold steel against my skin at night, aging our young bones by the minute. And the air was so crisp that we could take bites of the sweet dew before the morning sun scattered it. The hills were almost mountains and were named for their personalities. "Mount Motherfucker" lived across the road from our camp, and like many hills in the neighborhood, it had the ability to shoot sharp needles through your thighs, calves, and feet as you climbed it. Our barracks looked like a county jail—full of young men in boxers, card players, smokers, jokers, jailhouse lawyers, and fights.

The training offered us an advanced degree in aggression. It was one thousand times more intense than anything my brilliant high school football coaches asked us to do—obviously, we were there to learn combat, not plays. As a binger, I found it easy to replace food with aggression. I didn't realize the profound impact on my personality at the time, but MCT was one of my "Morpheus moments," and I was offered a choice between the blue pill (Sergeant Green) and the red pill of truth (Sergeant Sanchez). *I'll have an extra serving of the red pill, please!*

Sergeant Green represented everything that was clean and pure about the Marine Corps (if there was such a thing). His face resembled Steve Carell's, the actor/comedian from *The Office* and several funny movies, and his childlike enthusiasm for the innocent aspects of Marine culture were funny. Sergeant Green still used words that we were taught in boot camp. He called *sneakers* "go-fasters"; an *ink pen* was an "ink stick"; and a *poncho* was neatly referred to as a "burrito roll." Sergeant Green didn't sound off (yell); instead, he chatted in conversational tones with the platoon (group of Marines or other military units)—and this one was fifty guys deep. His uniform was crisp and creased; boots shined; his hair always cut close in the traditional "high and tight" (bald on the sides and back; small patch of very short hair on top); his face clean-shaven—similar to the drill instructors we'd just left. Sergeant Green lived by the book and didn't offer much room for improvisation. He was the blue pill; he was the status quo.

Sergeant Sanchez was the exact opposite. He was dark and gritty. He looked like George Lopez . . . without the jokes. Instead of innocent Marine vocabulary, Sanchez used spicier language. *Gear* was "trash"; *hands* were "dick skinners"; and young Marines were "motherfuckers." Sergeant Sanchez was intimidating, and he could stare you down with both eyes shut. He paced in front of the platoon like a warden on the catwalk, eyeballing everyone, frowning, and criticizing—pointing out errors with his index, pinkie, and thumb all at the same time. (For some reason, when pointing, Sanchez made the international fake pistol symbol with his index finger and thumb, except he then extended his pinky finger as the topper—like the "I love you" sign in sign language. I'm not sure why, but it was effectively memorable.) Sergeant Sanchez represented the darker side of the Marine Corps, the true purpose of why we were there and what we may be asked to do. He didn't sing; he didn't dance; he didn't smile. He believed Marines were made to break things and kill people. Sergeant Sanchez was the red pill. He was what I had been searching for my entire adolescent life, and I quickly and openly binged on his truth.

The choice between the two pills, between the two sergeants, was given to us on the first Sunday of the training cycle. I remember the exact moment. Sergeant Green had control of the platoon, and he gave us a speech about church. He talked about how God had saved him and how he was born again. It was like an alter call, a decisive moment, for sinners, lasting at least thirty minutes. Sergeant Green sat comfortably on an ammo can, reminiscing about his relationship with God as if he were talking to a dear old friend. Looking around, all I saw were fifty confused newbies.

Maybe he has a point? I wondered. "Jesus saves" was a big slogan in our church when I was a kid. *Maybe he means he can save us in combat?*

Either way, Sergeant Green was preaching.

Within the hour, control of the platoon was passed to Sergeant Sanchez. Once Green left the area, Sanchez called the platoon back to the deck and sat us down. "Get over here, motherfuckers!" The scowl on his face could intimidate Goliath. He looked as if he were about to go berserk and eat a baby—or the chaplain.

Sanchez paced slowly as all of us sat cross-legged on the concrete deck. "I heard you turds got a visit from the *Lord* today." Nobody said a peep, but our asses started to pray. "Let me tell you motherfuckers something." Sanchez's voice escalated while his boot heels clicked against the pavement. "I was on the ground when we liberated Kuwait. I fought in Iraq and I never saw *Jesus Christ* in the trenches, wearing a helmet and flak jacket, hookin' and jabbin' with the enemy. *Jesus* was nowhere to be found! Do you understand me?"

The air was so still that you could hear a pin drop. No one dared utter a sound. I expected a war-torn story of relying on your fellow Marines, your brothers, when in combat. Or some type of encouragement about teamwork and how we should rely on our training. We didn't get that one—not yet. All I could muster was an image of a bearded Jesus shadowboxing in a white robe covered by a bulletproof vest.

Sanchez continued to sound off as his black eyebrows formed a sharp V shape between his beady eyes. "The only one I saw out there in the desert was the *devil*. That's right—the *devil*! If you want to give your heart to something, you give it to the *devil*. War is not nice. War will make you drink blood and piss sand. Do you hear me, motherfuckers?"

I was shocked, stunned, silenced, to say the least. *Could he really worship the devil?* I grew up believing that most Latinos were Catholic, but this guy took a sharp right turn down a road we didn't expect. Sanchez stopped his slow pacing, landing square in front of the platoon. He pointed at himself with three fingers and said, "Yeah, that's right: I worship the devil. If you want to follow that other shit, pack your *trash* and take your pussy-ass out of my platoon!"

And that was it—for now. That was our choice: blue pill or red pill, Jesus or the devil, Sergeant Green or Sergeant Sanchez. Sergeant Green's brand of the Marine Corps offered little satisfaction to the newly titled Marine—especially me, a binger looking for a new obsession. None of us expected devil worship, but I think we realized what Sanchez was trying to say. Or I did anyway. I joined the Marines for Sanchez's version, for his type of validation. He could show me the way. He could teach me the truth.

Sergeant Sanchez didn't waste any time establishing his leadership philosophy with us. The next day, after hiking into the field and establishing camp for the week, we were left alone to practice our weapons training. It was one of those quiet moments where the instructors left us alone for hours. They taught us how to disassemble, clean, and reassemble the M249 SAW machine gun. They had us do it all afternoon. Take it apart, put it together, and take it apart again . . . and again . . . and again. The next day, we were all going to be timed in the drill. If you did it too slow, you didn't pass that series of instruction and something bad would likely happen.

Our platoon was lined up out in an open field in the hills of Pendleton, like nice neat rows of corn. All of us sat in the dirt, equally spaced out with our weapons in front of us. Take it apart, put it together, take it apart, and put it together. We were in the hot sun for hours while Sergeant Sanchez and the other troop handlers sat in a tent in the not-so-far distance. After several hours, Sanchez appeared and slowly paced through our rows with his prison warden walk. "Listen up, third!" (We were "third platoon"— when addressing the group, you're often referred to, collectively, as "third.") "I'm going to find out which of you motherfuckers have been sleeping. Some of you out here have been wasting your time and don't know how to put this weapon together. Trust me. I'm going to find you." Asses puckered as he stalked.

Sanchez walked past me and stopped at the Marine a few down the line. "Go ahead, boy," he commanded. The kid froze in place and started to fumble with the parts. The barrel dropped on the ground at least three times as he tried to beat the clock. "What's the matter, motherfucker? You're the one, aren't you?" The kid was all thumbs; the spring mechanism shot across the ground in front of me. "You're going to need that," Sanchez barked as he lifted a boot and stomped the kid square in the chest.

"Stand up, *shit bird*." Sanchez scowled as he impatiently jerked the kid up to his feet by the collar.

"What's the matter with you, motherfucker?" Sanchez slapped the Marine's mouth. "I just taught you this. Give me your ID card!" Another stiff slap followed—*smack!* The rest of the Marines sat quietly as Sergeant Sanchez patrolled the ranks. In total, he collected five or six ID cards, delivering smacks to each of the sleepers. Everyone knew to pay attention after that; I know I did. His lessons could save our lives . . . and save us from getting fat lips.

That night after chow (dinner), Sergeant Sanchez gave us another speech. He started out calm but firm. It felt as if we were all by a campfire, and I thought he was finally going to let his guard down and level with us as men. "Marines, I know some of you didn't like what I did today," he acknowledged in a low tone. "We're all Marines, and we should conduct ourselves as such—even me."

Okay, I thought, waiting for his real truth to show itself.

"But this is my fucking platoon! If you don't like the way I run it, too bad!"

Great. At least we know where he stands.

Sergeant Sanchez continued to lather. "Better yet, if you think you can kick my ass . . . I'll let you lead this platoon." He was on his feet now, pointing at himself with the *I love you* sign. "I'll take my chevrons [rank insignia worn on the collar] off right now. Meet me at the tree line and we'll fight for the guidon [flag]. Whoever comes back with it is the leader. Good to go . . . ? I said, 'Good to go, motherfuckers?'!"

Sanchez continued to pace and point like a raged lion. He seemed serious too. Nobody stood to accept his challenge, but something told me that he would fight anybody who did. He was our leader—he was salty, experienced, and had been to war. Maybe he had killed people; perhaps he wanted to kill us. Either way, the red pill was digesting, and I was bingeing on it.

If he didn't have the full command and respect of the platoon before that moment, he definitely had it now. In a short time, we learned that he worshiped the devil; he didn't mind smacking young motherfuckers—I mean, Marines—around; and he would gladly give up his leadership spot if one of us could beat him up. This was outside the lines, beyond the boundaries that we thought existed in training. Sergeant Sanchez pushed those limits, and now we were operating in some type of primal tribe—like *Lord of the Flies*. We were his, and he wanted us to be like him. He wanted us to be cagey, fierce, fearless war fighters. His brand of the truth rushed through our platoon like a tornado. Those who feared him listened to him. Those who listened to him wanted to be like him. We mimicked his speech, his points, and his attitude toward everything.

We were different when we returned to the barracks a week later—confident, assured, arrogant, cocky; no longer "green recruits. Before we hit the showers, each platoon was taken to the armory to clean our weapons and turn them in. Our platoon, the third platoon, presented its new identity the minute we arrived at the cleaning tables.

First platoon occupied the tables next to us. Both platoons were now situated close to each other. One hundred men occupied ten cleaning tables in the yard for several hours, which produced many icy and tense moments. Mainly because they didn't like us (who knew what brand of the Marine's they were being taught) and we were better than them (lessons straight from our leader). Shoving matches started with little provocation, and guys squared off more than they cleaned. A bad stare, a cross eye, or a visual dismissal would start the "motherfucker wars." The aggressive tension blanketed the yard, and after a short time, guys from our two platoons were itching to fight each other over nothing.

Before a rumble could break out, Sergeant Sanchez stepped in to calm everyone down. He paced over to the tables with his three-finger point at the ready. "The next motherfucker that starts a fight will have to answer to me personally. Do you animals understand that?"

Grumbles could be heard from both platoons. "Aye, Sergeant."

"And, third—don't let me catch you backing down from one of these first faggots or we'll meet at the tree line."

Well, that cleared things up.

Sanchez's mixed message squealed like a loud dog whistle in the pound. Eyes darted around the armory, looking for negative contact, frowns, and signs of disrespect. "Fuck you" and "Eat me" echoed across the cleaning tables. Suddenly, I noticed a sharp movement to my right. I dropped my cleaning gear and squared myself toward their table just in time to see Private Devine, the scrawniest guy in our platoon, swing a machine gun barrel at the back shoulder blades of Private Geiger, the biggest redneck in first platoon. *Crack!*

Geiger was so corn-fed and amped on adrenaline that he merely dropped to one knee. I thought it would've crumpled him, but Devine didn't pack that much power. I looked over at Sergeant Sanchez and saw him mouth to another troop handler from first platoon, "Did you see that? That motherfucker hit him with a sixty barrel!" The platoons were quickly separated after that, and the feud (the war) had begun. Sergeant Sanchez elected *first* platoon our *first* real enemy. *Priceless!*

We had many little skirmishes with first platoon over the next few weeks. We didn't get to interact with them much over the course of the month, except when we would come back in from the field. We would see them at the chow hall or back at the camp. Their barracks were adjacent to ours. Shoving matches persisted, and dirty names were thrown across the yard like naval gunfire. "Your sister's a whore—did I ever tell you that?" was a light insult in this crowd.

Looking back, our feud with first platoon was as deliberate as the nose on my face. It was also like a fire that was being stoked for a month, getting hotter and hotter with each poke of the coals . . . or with each encounter. Sergeant Sanchez never let us get too close, but he didn't let us get too far away from them either. We were like a pack of hungry lions staring at a herd of female water buffalos every time they got near us—until the last two days of the training cycle.

The last two days of MCT were scheduled to be "administrative" days. We had been in the field for the majority of the month. All we had to do now was return our gear to the supply warehouse and get our orders. I was headed to intelligence training in Virginia. (*Military intelligence*—I know, I know. After all that fat, after all that starving, I was still going to be an oxymoron . . . Very funny!)

Still, once our gear was turned in and our weapons were cleaned for the last time, Sergeant Sanchez decided to test our resolve.

"Left, right, left . . . Left, right, left!" Sanchez shouted out the cadence while we marched down the road away from the supply warehouse. I could see the guys from first platoon in the short distance. They were standing in formation (nice neat rows/ranks) on the side of the road, apparently waiting for something. As we approached and passed their formation I heard, "Column—left. March!"

He can't be serious . . .

Of course, we obeyed.

Yes, as we marched past first platoon, Sergeant Sanchez tested our resolve. His command "column left" meant "take a left turn"—directly into first platoon's formation. Steering us into them was like steering an eighteen-wheeler into a parked bus—not a great idea. The result was worse than a car wreck. This was known as "breaking ranks," and it was a slap in the face . . . a challenge . . . a duel. It was fighting words for all involved.

The fight was started the second we violated first platoon's ranks. We marched through their platoon like a silverback gorilla looking to mark its territory. "What the fuck!" someone yelled as the pushing and shoving led to many left jabs and right crosses.

"Get out of there, Marines!" Sergeant Sanchez bellowed as he grabbed us by the collars, throwing us in a heap to the other side of the road. "You want a piece of them, third?"

"Aye, Sergeant!" we crowed as a group.

Sanchez trotted over to first platoon's troop handlers and started talking to their sergeant. We stood in formation, huffing and puffing, waiting for him to come back. "We're going to kill those guys," someone said. I glanced over, and it didn't look as if Sanchez was killing anybody. His chat was hardly an argument. It looked more like a drug deal. The two sergeants stood close together, nodding, fist bumping, and even smiling a little. Eventually they nodded their heads at the same time, and Sanchez literally sprinted back across the road to where he left us.

He smirked. "You ready, third?"

"Aye, Sergeant . . . They suck . . . I'm gonna fuck someone up!" the guys roared at will.

Sanchez quickly took his spot at the front of the platoon. "You got your chance, third. Follow me and remember: stay away from the groin and the eyes. Anything else is fair game!"

With that, Sanchez took us across the dirt road that led up a small hill. First platoon followed at a safe distance. At the top sat a grassy knoll that was surrounded on three sides by steeper hills. Both platoons were isolated now. Our presence wasn't visible by anyone in the camp below, and I knew we had arrived. This area looked like a natural MMA octagon—like a cage—and it was the place we were going to finally do real battle for the first time. With third platoon (us) on one side, and first platoon (them) on the other, Sergeant Sanchez stood in the middle of the knoll and said: "Listen up! If anyone asks, this is called 'Bull in the ring.' Stay away from the groin and the eyes. Everything else is fair game!" Sanchez quickly retreated from the knoll.

The two platoons rushed each other like the scene from *Braveheart* when the Scottish ran across the battlefield to fight the English. Bodies clashed and heads butted as one hundred bloodthirsty Marines finally got to face off. We all had opponents, someone we could wrestle, punch, choke, rip, and dominate. I first saw Geiger (the big corn-fed redneck who got hit with a machine gun barrel) find Devine (the small guy who swung the barrel), and I assumed Devine was a goner. I'm not sure what happened after that. I located an opponent I didn't know, and we tangled: wrestled, punched, choked, and ripped. I'm pretty sure I dominated. Guys bumped into each other in the melee. I threw body blow after body blow. *Ooof!* I got punched in the face, and I punched other guys in the face. It was a rumble, and I might have even punched my own squad leader before I realized that we were on the same side. Somehow I ended up on the ground in the dirt when the fight ended. I had a guy from first platoon in a choke hold, while another guy from first platoon had me in a headlock.

(Okay, so the "sleeper hold" was still my best move even after all that combat training. I couldn't resist slapping on the sleeper after watching so much professional wrestling—WWF—as a kid. Hulkamania was runnin' wild in the grassy knoll that day, brother!)

The sergeants broke up each skirmish and separated everyone. We stood there huffing and puffing, proud of what just happened. I glanced across the knoll and saw that first platoon was beat up. They had black eyes, bloody noses, scratches, and even a few rips in their T-shirts. It was like looking in the mirror as they stared back at us, checking out their handiwork.

As we marched down the dirt road back to camp, I felt extreme pride (the deadly sin kind). I was so far away from the fat kid—from the obese guy I had been the year before. I was now cagey, a fighter, and ready to eat raw meat before pouncing at anyone I thought was unjust. I wasn't bingeing on food anymore. No. Now I was bingeing on another poison that I couldn't see, and that was much more dangerous than I could imagine.

With my red pill completely digested, it was time to say good-bye to MCT and to Sergeant Sanchez. The next day, our platoon stood in formation as the battalion commander (head cheese) read the graduation commencement. What a sight that must have been. Two of his platoons—first (them) and third (us)—standing at attention with black eyes and fat lips. Lucky for me, I escaped with a few scratches on my arm and some red marks on my neck. The commander must have wondered why we looked so rough, but the odds were good that he knew already.

After the ceremony, a buddy and I walked up to Sergeant Sanchez to say good-bye. It felt a little strange because none of us had really ever had a meaningful one-on-one conversation with him before. Over the previous month, he talked, and we listened; he threatened, and we shit our pants. Still, my friend and I wanted closure and felt like thanking him for the training and wishing him well. "Hey, Pedersen—nice job out there! You too, Rubberford." (My buddy's name was "Rutherford," but Sanchez always dicked it up.) "You motherfuckers take care!"

And that was it. There wasn't much more to say. There wasn't much more that he needed to say. Sanchez strengthened my backbone and gave me my first enemy. Obesity wasn't my enemy now. I didn't even know that "Doug" anymore—no one did. I didn't think about my childhood for a second after that. Not about being fat, being teased, or being a binge-eating quitter. No. Now I was bingeing on aggression, testosterone, and competition. Looking back, arrogance was an easy replacement for fear and food. Instead of being a binge eater, I was bingeing on my quest for significance—silently judging others and being competitive, narcissistic, and arrogant—and I cultivated a general sense of self-superiority within myself (and wrongfully so).

How was I to know? I was mentally ready to break things and kill people, just like Sanchez. I was aggressive, quick to anger, slow to smile. His red pill of truth tasted like sweet syrup to a binger like me. I pointed with the *I love you* sign, and I adopted several new philosophies:

- It's better to swim with the sharks than to float with the bait.
- If the Marines wanted me to have a wife, they would have issued me one.
- Survival of the fittest is real.
- You just can't kill me!

Four years later, I was sent back to Camp Pendleton to serve with the Second Battalion, Fifth Marines—with the infantry and with "Rubberford," my buddy from MCT. I was salty by then, having earned several achievement medals, a noncommissioned officer rank (corporal), and having been deployed overseas for a year. Sure enough, and much to my surprise, Sanchez was already stationed with that unit. He had returned to the fleet (regular Marine Corps) after completing several years at his training assignment (MCT).

Sanchez remembered the others and me from third platoon. We laughed and reminisced about the old days. He remembered Sergeant Green and the devil speech. I learned that it was an orchestrated event that he and Green did with every training cycle. It was their way of passing the time and motivating young trainees with squishy minds. Their job was to teach us to fight and to put our minds in that dark place—to give us the red pill and teach us the truth. I asked him if he regretted anything he did while training young Marines or if he'd ever been confronted once he got back to the fleet. Sanchez looked me in the eye and only had one thing to say: "I regret swearing so much. My three-year-old son jumped into my bed last night and said, 'Good night, motherfucker!'"

CHAPTER 7

ARROGANCE ISN'T BLISS

ar·ro·gant

adjective

1. *: exaggerating or disposed to exaggerate one's own worth or importance often by an overbearing manner*
2. *: showing an offensive attitude of superiority*

—Merriam-Webster

I don't know about you, but there was a time when I felt I was the best person in the room. Not that anyone ever told me so. It's just that since I got skinny and became a Marine there were many instances where I truly believed that I was special—the toughest guy, the fastest runner, the most handsome, and even the smartest guy with the most common sense. Now, I'm not saying that I literally walked around with my nose in the air, insulting everyone around me. However, if people knew what I was really thinking much of the time, that's probably the image they would get. I suppose you could say that I was a bit arrogant when it came to relating to other people.

To me, I was just finally demonstrating my pride (deadly sin kind) about winning in life. Perhaps like a prizefighter that's competed for the title. Mike Tyson had to slug it out with guys like Larry Holmes and Michael Spinks to be considered the best. He had to beat up thirty men before he was called a world champion—something most men haven't done or wouldn't try. In my case, I believed that I had knocked out obesity with one punch, on the first try. I volunteered for the toughest, most respected fighting force in the world, and I excelled at it. I accomplished something (*finally!*) that not many fat kids did in 1993. I believed that I was a special somebody now (in my mind at least)—no longer an oxymoron, no longer weak, disrespected, or irrelevant.

Was this irony? Well, it definitely wasn't the kind of irony we find gently funny at times. Like if you consider why number 2 pencils are "number two" when everybody uses them kind of ironic. Or when you realize that a choking Smurf still turns blue type of ironic. No, not that gently funny. No. After a few years in the Marine Corps, and at the ripe old age of twenty-two, I couldn't see the irony in my story. There was nothing gently funny about how I grew out of being a lazy, insecure kid into an overactive, overconfident, and silently arrogant jerk. But I suppose it is ironic how my same human need, my same lust, for certainty and significance that drove my obesity had turned me into this new, still heavily flawed direction.

Since becoming a Marine my new binge, my new obsession, craved grunt life. The word "grunt" dates back to the World War II—era Marines. *Grunts* were the infantrymen—the guys with rifles . . . the guys who did the fighting. If you looked the word up in the Urban Dictionary, you would find this:

Grunt is an acronym used during WW2 for troops who had no formal training, or skills. G-general, R-replacement, UNT-untrained, . . . GRUNT, as they had no special training, they were given rifles and sent to the front.

Grunts do all the fighting.

Or:

The term "grunt" is used in the military as a general term for someone [whose] MOS (Military Occupational Specialty) is "Infantry" . . . . The opposite of a "grunt" is a "pougue," which is a derogatory reference to pretty much anyone who isn't a grunt, but normally reserved for Marines who work in an office or some other rear-echelon job as part of their regular duties ("In the rear with the gear").

If you ain't a grunt you ain't SHIT!

Bingeing on grunt life was a no-brainer for me. It virtually erased the "fat quitter" image I carried of myself as a teenager while still satisfying my chase for significance. It was so important to be like and relate to Louie—and to the invincible grunt image that Sergeant Sanchez portrayed at MCT. Everything I had learned in my first six months of being a Marine made me believe that going to the grunts was the toughest, hardest, most dangerous road for an enlisted guy like me—and I just had to get there.

Before being assigned to the grunts, the Marines were going to make me a military intelligence specialist (still an oxymoron—and I was actually going to attend a formal school to become one. Gently funny, I know). It had been a while since my recruiter had me read the job description, but he explained that the Intel guys were responsible for the "collection, integration, analysis, and distribution of intelligence." In my mind, that meant that I would spy on someone, look at other information from other spies, make a WAG (wild-ass guess) about what the information meant, and then tell the boss.

After MCT, they sent me to a Navy base in Dam Neck, Virginia— home of the Naval and Marine Intelligence Training Center (NMITC). *Dam Neck* didn't sound too intelligent, but I quickly learned that it was easy duty for us newly titled Marines, mainly because Dam Neck was more like a community college than an elite spy incubator. It was nestled in the "lush" coastal swamp outside Virginia Beach. The base E-Club (enlisted bar) was the most popular spot. It was called The Shifting Sands Beach Club, and they didn't check anyone's age. The Navy trainees lived in hotel-style two-man rooms that reminded me more of dorms than traditional military barracks. Instead of field training, we went to class all day. There were administration buildings, cars in parking lots, sidewalks, and tons of young sailors carrying their training materials. Intel training was about the classroom; it was school. Instead of bowel movements in the dirt, Marine intelligence focused on spitballs through a straw.

Even though we (thirty of us Marines) were the minority on this base, we felt as if we were men among boys. Young sailors didn't have any context to what young Marines were or the training we had already gone through—I thought. Call it an "inner-service rivalry"; call it a "feud"; call it what you will. We called them squids, and they called us jarheads. It didn't bother me one bit. I was proud to be called a jarhead; I had earned it. We wore green woodland camouflage uniforms with jet-black combat boots. They wore white Cracker Jack—style uniforms with bibs around their necks and *dog dishes* on their heads. *Make fun of my hat, will you!* When sailors weren't wearing their Elvis impersonator suits with baby bibs, they wore baby-blue button-down shirts with dark blue bell-bottom pants, boots called "boondockers," and the traditional white dog dish hat. *Bow wow!* They looked like janitors; we looked like warriors.

You would expect Marines to feel superior to sailors. It was in our DNA, and we treated them as if they were our annoying siblings. It was May 1994 by now. I was twenty years old, and I couldn't help projecting my competitive arrogance toward the people I was closest to—my fellow Marines. Sure, the word "intelligence" was thrown around a lot, but we were all still young men with sharp egos and type A personalities, not to mention incapable of growing beards. We were a primal tribe, and I imagine that the thirty of us in the Marine Intel class were just like any college freshman fraternity. *Go Greek or go home!*

My feelings of superiority started to change after one of our first free weekends. I didn't assume too much about anyone before that (and I made a few solid friends), but things changed when our class decided to get wasted together—you know: drunk, intoxicated, blitzed, sauced, three sheets to the wind, assed out. I learned much later that Japanese businessmen believe that you can't truly know or trust a person until you've been *assed out* together—that was the easy rumor to believe in my twenties. The theory made sense, though, because you can presumably see a drunken person's true colors: angry, sad, honest, happy, mean, smart, or just plain dumb.

Day drinking at that time might have been dumb, but it sure made sense to the thirty of us. Without incriminating too many of these guys, let's just say that all of us acted like fools at some point, with varying degrees of drunken stupidity. During that weekend, I watched as a grown man peed his pants while sitting in our gazebo—fully awake, drunk, and laughing the whole time (okay, we dared him to do it). Another guy tried to sprint across the grass field outside our barracks to fight three sailors he didn't even know. He was so drunk that he couldn't stand up straight, let alone run straight or talk straight. He managed to blurt out, "I'm . . .

going to . . . kick your . . . Cracker Jack . . . asses!" before he collapsed like a folding chair after his fifth step. I told you: men among boys.

Not to be topped, however, the second-to-biggest fool turned out to be the guy assigned to "fire watch." He was the one of us assigned to be the uniformed sentry, the guy who stood guard duty in our barracks, the guy who was supposed to log incidents and mischief for the day: fire watch. Anyway, he drank so much (while on duty) that he passed out on the couch in our TV lounge. *Snoooorrrre!* In no time at all, a gang of us worked faster than Jimmie Johnson's pit crew to toilet paper him to the couch, laughing and giggling the whole time. *Yuk-yuk-yuk . . . Tee-hee, tee-hee!* We encased him in toilet paper so that only his head and face were exposed. *He looks like King Tut's mummy! Get the hot dogs . . .*

With shameless pride, guys grabbed their cameras to take novelty (blackmail) shots. An anonymous prankster then grabbed an uncooked hot dog from the fridge and dipped one end into the mayonnaise jar. Once it was loaded, the prankster gently poked, probed, rubbed, and wiped the sleeping fire watch's lips, nose, and mouth with it. I never laughed harder the whole time I was there. *Cackle . . . snicker!* The fire watch never took the hot dog like a pacifier, but that was the goal. *Click!*

Our class was forced to sober up that weekend when the biggest fool decided to roll over in his sleep. This wouldn't have been a big deal except that he was on the edge of his top rack (bed) in the squad bay. After a drunken snore, the he rolled right off his bed and dropped six feet, like a sack of potatoes, to the hard tile floor. *Thud!* He was knocked unconscious (not that he was awake before it happened), and he had split his head wide open. Blood spilled out of his head like red Kool-Aid, right before everything he ate and drank that day launched from the pit of his belly and out of his mouth, onto the freshly waxed and buffed floor. *Wretch!*

We had to call the adults after that. The base paramedics took him to the hospital. The doctors pumped his stomach like a well in order to treat his alcohol poisoning; he was in the hospital for four days. When he got back to the barracks, his head was wrapped tightly in white medical bandages, like the guy/couch we toilet papered. At least no one put a happy ending hot dog near his lips and snapped pictures while he lay helpless on the deck.

I had my own set of adventures that weekend. My drink of choice came straight out of a bottle of Wild Turkey. Of course, I acted like a wild turkey, but I kept my pee in the toilet, no one put a hot dog pacifier near my face, and I didn't head butt the floor. My sole purpose was to hang out all day drinking, daring, and goading before going to the Shifting Sands to do my rendition of the Samoan jackhammer. After just the right amount of dancing, I looked to play a common version of "I'll show you mine if you show me yours" with one of the many waves (female sailors) who crashed around our barracks. It was simple for me: I wanted to get laid. If a Japanese businessman was in our group, he would likely conclude that I was a wild turkey in heat.

It was easy for me to think less of many of the guys after that. They acted foolish, and even though I did as well, I judged them for it. I'd sacrificed everything I knew to get into the Marines, and I wanted to be the best. I was the guy who studied hard at night; I trained my body hard during the day; I made flash cards to take with me; and I wanted to be taken seriously as a Marine and as an Intel professional. So instead of trying to fit in the pack, I made it my job to quietly mess with them. One of my good buddies was an older guy who had been a cop before joining the Marines. He pulled pranks because he was a practical joker. I joined him because I liked him and thought that many of the guys deserved it.

The ketchup and mustard caper was my absolute favorite, though. As it turned out, my friend and I were assigned to clean the head (bathroom) every morning, which meant that we had to sweep, mop, and scrub the place. Ours looked like a typical locker room-style bathroom: open showers, urinals, and a row of eight or nine toilets. *Hey, guy, pass the sports section, would ya?* This job sucked, so while I received my master's degree in janitorial work, we passed the time by setting ketchup and mustard traps at night. It required patience and skill—and it felt like setting traps for wild turkeys. Our targets were the unsuspecting drunks who would come in during the middle of the night to drain their bladders before passing out in their beds.

The trap required one plastic packet of ketchup (like the ones you get with your fries) and one plastic packet of mustard (like the ones that *should* go with a Dodger Dog). To set the trap, we folded each packet in half and placed the ketchup at "three o'clock" and the mustard at "nine o'clock" on the white porcelain toilet rim. To complete the operation, we simply (and gently) closed the U-shaped toilet seat to keep the packets folded and pressurized.

Without fail, a drunk or sleepy Marine would stumble into the dark toilet room and plop down on the trap seat. The second he did, the ketchup and mustard exploded like a landmine, spraying bursts of red and yellow goop on the guy's unsuspecting butt cheeks and testicle region. *Dammit!* The next morning, we would check our traps to see if one hit. My sides would split every time we saw a trail of red and yellow footprints headed straight into the shower room. *Morons!*

After six months of wild turkey action in Dam Neck, I was ready for the fleet (active Marine units). I had graduated Intel school with top honors and was the only junior enlisted guy to be recognized in front of the class by our trainers. They even presented me with a certificate, proving how smart I really was. I didn't need their validation, though. I already believed that I was the best: there weren't any ketchup or mustard bombs on *my* nuts. *If Mrs. Magnolia could only see me now—damn hippie!*

Much to my disappointment, I wasn't sent to the grunts after Intel school. Instead, I was sent to Marine Aircraft Group 12 (MAG-12, or just MAG) in Iwakuni, Japan. I stayed positive and excited to deploy overseas, but deep down I really hated the MAG. It was a "pougue" assignment. MAG was on an air base; it was the "Air Wing," or just the "Wing." A long concrete airstrip was the centerpiece of this base. There were no hills, no grass, no trees, and no grunts, which limited my opportunity to binge on aggression.

Pilots were the real war fighters in this unit, and F/A-18 Hornets (fighter jets) were the weapon of choice. It wasn't quite like *Top Gun*, unless you were a "fighter jock." Instead of call signs like Maverick, Goose, Iceman, and Hollywood, these guys had names like Chugger, Hogg, and Shag. The enlisted guys (like me) didn't have call signs, unless you consider "support" a call sign. I sure didn't. Support had tire gauges and potbellies; support pumped gas and washed windows. I saw MAG as one big gas station, just like the one I worked at in high school.

I didn't try to fit in there at all, for the Wing was known for being soft, especially for the enlisted men like me. What bothered me the most was that I saw seasoned Marines who wanted to be soft. In fact, they enjoyed it; they liked the easy lifestyle, away from the hardness of the groundside—like my new boss, a master sergeant. He was a far cry from the example that Sergeant Sanchez set for me earlier that year. The master sergeant was short and looked like Moe from the Three Stooges (same haircut and everything—not Marine Corps regulation . . . *Nyuk, nyuk, nyuk*). He told me once, "I'm on the ROAD program. You know: R-etire O-n A-ctive D-uty?" This was not inspiring to a young hardcore like me. I thought he was nasty from day one.

My officer in charge (big boss) wasn't any better. He was a lieutenant colonel and intelligence officer. He came from a war college in Washington, DC, and had spent most of his life in think tanks—not real tanks, I figured. With his wire-framed glasses, mousy face, and neatly parted silver hair, he looked more like the main character from *The Nutty Professor* than the hard-charging balls of steel colonel that Jack Nicholson played in *A Few Good Men*. "You need me on the wall! You want me on the wall! You can't handle the truth!"

The guy that I focused all my competitive aggression toward, however, was my roommate. To me, his name sounded like "Doofus," and that's how I always thought of him. He was only senior to me by six months, but he always wanted to exert his authority (new Marine reflex, I suppose). He was taller than I was, but his oil-speckled glasses, long red hair (for Marine standards), wrinkled uniform, and Hershey Bar-polished boots wouldn't let me respect him. I believed he was a dirtbag of a Marine, a waste of space and good oxygen. Doofus didn't want to train hard (run, do sit-ups, practice the obstacle course, or climb the ropes). He would rather whine and complain: "This sucks! I should be an officer right now. My recruiter screwed me over. I'm getting out!" *Blah, blah, blah.*

I couldn't have cared less about his plight. The more time we spent together (we worked in the same shop and lived in the same barracks room—*just the two of us . . . you and I . . .*), the more agitated I got with him. I figured that his recruiter had done him a favor and had done me a disservice. When he wanted to take shortcuts at work, I wanted to expose and upstage him. When he wanted to fall out of unit runs and act like a weak pussy, I literally wanted to walk circles around him. When he wanted to hang out, I did everything but. When he ditched field day (weekly cleaning), I wanted to fight him. I thought he should have been in the band, not in the Marine Corps. Somehow I was perfect; somehow he was a turd.

My proof that I was better than Doofus came when I was sent to Thailand later that year. I was the only one from our Intel shop sent to represent our unit during a massive regional training exercise—Cobra Gold '95. The Marines, Navy, and Air Force were participating; so were the Thais and the Australians—maybe ten thousand participants at one point. Doofus didn't get selected. He wasn't sent to Australia or Korea (as I was), and I concluded that I must be better than him. I had to be. Without war, all we (I) had were deployments to far-off lands and training to elevate our (my) status. Somewhere during those five weeks, I grew further out of my britches—and sold them to a Thai colonel.

Five weeks in Thailand as a young twenty-year-old Marine was like winning the Mega Millions drawing. Suddenly, I had everything at my disposal: money (the dollar was strong then), girls, alcohol, and luxury hotel living (according to Thai standards). Life in Thailand was rich in comparison to the milquetoast existence that I believed Japan had to offer. "Anything went" in Thailand—like Las Vegas on steroids. I felt like a king, and it was the only time in my six years of service that I ever considered deserting. I was far from being homesick. I couldn't think of anyone but myself, forgetting my family and friends as well as the obese couch potato that had long passed.

I hung out with a few buddies from the unit that I could actually tolerate. Jim worked in the operations shop; Ben (no relation) worked in the administration shop. We stayed on a remote and rustic Thai Marine base near the coast. Tropical beaches littered with wild sand grass and short palm trees separated the Gulf of Thailand from the open dirt fields and shanty Thai villagers who lived nearby. The real perk, however, was the twenty-minute *tuk-tuk* (Thai taxi) ride to Pattaya Beach.

As we knew it, Pattaya Beach was the biggest red-light district in the world. Ben, Jim, and I tried to ease into the scene, but it was almost impossible to go slow. Of course, we made it our job to visit the long strip of bars as early and as often as we could—and we never missed a day or night in Pattaya in five weeks of the deployment. The bar district looked like Mardi Gras every day. Everything was for sale and was negotiable: watches, clothes, jewelry, and mystery meat. Streetwalkers littered the streets: women looking for young men, and young men looking for young men. Thai boxing rings were set up like peep shows, and exotic parrots, boa constrictors, and lizards were available for photos (or anything else, I'm sure). Alcohol flowed like the mighty Mississippi. Instead of pool tables, every bar had dancing girls who specialized in the most disturbing stripper tricks that you just don't see in the good old U S of A.

The first woman who spoke to me actually had good English skills. She stood next to our table, dancing in place with a full-lipped white toothy smile. "What's your name?"

Each of us grabbed our beers and took a quick swig. "Franklin Johnson. What's yours?" For some reason, I didn't want to give her my real name, as if she would enter me in the national Thai database or something.

My new friend didn't reply—at least not with spoken words. No, this nice local decided to reply in the written form. She backed up several feet from our table, revealing her naked body, and knelt to the floor, gripping a black Sharpie marker with her hoo-ha (yes, with her lady business, kitty, yum yum, honey pot, lady garden). None of us knew what to expect; our attention was locked squarely on the Sharpie. *Hmmmm?* She crouched down on all fours and carefully scribed the following message (in cursive) on a piece of white construction paper that was delicately positioned on the dance floor beneath her hips: *Welcome to Pattaya Beach, Franklin Johnson!* Impressive—not a single typo!

Thailand was insane. It was Caligula's last orgy and far away from *Doofus* and the rest of the nastiness back home at the MAG. It was overkill, but when you're a twenty-year-old Marine (or maybe just a guy in general), you can't look away, even when the stripper tricks get downright disturbing. I saw one of them huff with her muff and launch a sharp needle dart from a two-foot bamboo pipe to pop a balloon that was six feet away. Another pushed out several Ping-Pong balls into a glass of water—like a chicken laying eggs—while another girl popped the cap off a Coke bottle (non-twist off . . . *Coke is it!*). Still a few others pulled strand after strand of roses, razor blades, and needles from their vajayjays, like a magician pulling long, colorful scarves out of a magic hat. *WTF, dude?*

Despite all the good life I was getting, it was a riot in the streets that gave me the most status. It happened several weeks into the deployment. Jim, Ben, and I were sitting at our favorite table, feeling like locals in the biggest go-go bar ever: Caligula. Karaoke music was playing in the background. We had just returned from the stage after singing our rendition of the Eagles' "Hotel California" (that song played several times per night, and we loved to sing along every time). Then out of the crowds, a frenzy of people in the streets started to swarm like hornets.

"*Fight* at the Marine Disco!" someone yelled out. None of us knew what it was, but we rushed toward the center of the storm. Hundreds of Thais littered the streets in some type of revolt . . . or flash mob of locals that were upset about something. Violent pushing and shoving started, and I felt as if I were back in the grassy knoll at MCT. I started a rampage, punching anyone in sight. *It's better to swim with the sharks than to float with the bait,* my instincts told me. All I wanted to do was fight my way through the crowd and get into an opening. So I rushed through them like an NFL running back. Chairs, clothes, and heads of lettuce flew through the air like geese heading south for the winter. Thai men yelled in anger while the women screamed, in general, defending themselves with needles and razor blades, I imagined.

I finally fought through the massive crowds, causing as much damage as I could, and found a clearing at the end of the strip. Jim was there, but he wasn't in good shape. He was sitting on the curb in front of an abandoned bar holding his face. Several sailors hovered over him. I ran over to them and Jim nodded his head at me. *Great—he's alive!* He mumbled a few words, but he couldn't speak. Jim got hit in the face with a beer bottle; his party was over. Jim was sent back to Japan the next day to get his broken jaw wired shut.

While we tended to Jim, Ben stumbled into the clearing. *Great—he's alive too!* Ben had his huge northeastern grin plastered across his face. He looked like the Cheshire cat—or as if he ate the Cheshire Cat. He was holding the back of his head, but he had no recognition as to what was going on with it. We sat him down and saw a huge cut. It looked like he had been split with a small ax. He mumbled something about getting hit in the head with a piano leg, and I had to laugh out loud. *Chair leg, table leg, rooster leg—sure. Piano leg? Hmmm?*

Anyway, Ben got thirty-five stitches in his head, but he was able to stay. He wasn't completely out of the woods because for the next month he had to explain to every officer he passed why he wasn't wearing his cover (hat) outside—a big no no . . . *Too funny!*

As for me . . . *Well, you just can't kill me*, I thought. I didn't have a scratch on me. It was as if I were blessed or something. I don't know how, but I dodged that bullet too. This confidence tasted like sweet syrup to a binger like me. I got off on it, and Doofus and everyone like him had no chance of penetrating my arrogance after that. How could they? I had a business (selling uniforms I could scrounge up to the Thai Marines), I had a house (living in the Royal Thai Hotel every chance I got), I was popular (threw parties as if I were Hugh Hefner himself), and I was invincible (proven by the riot). I was perfect; they (the whole Wing) were turds.

My year in Japan was over a few months later. It was bittersweet because I was finally leaving the gas station for an assignment back at Camp Pendleton, California, where the grunts lived and trained (remember MCT?). You would think that my attitude toward my fellow Marines would change once I shipped out, but my tunnel vision continued to narrow over the next year as I spiraled deeper into my arrogant (and now negative) attitude.

Much to my dismay, the powers that controlled my destiny at the time did not send me to the grunts—still! Despite my best efforts to volunteer, trade, and take anything grunt related, they sent me to an artillery unit: the Cannon Cockers. I wasn't terribly excited about this assignment either, but at least the enlisted guys (like me) were the war fighters; they were outside a lot instead of in offices. But in the end, I still felt held back from my strong urge to be at the front with the grunts. The Cannon Cockers weren't at the front lines. They didn't hump (walk or hike all over the place with heavy backpacks)—they drove everywhere! Their motto: "If you can't truck it, fuck it!" *Great! Instead of the real grunts, they sent me to the fake grunts.* This wasn't good enough for an arrogant binger like me. I needed to suffer; I needed the real thing. Somehow I became Lieutenant Dan: "Goddamn it, [Gump]!" What are you doing? You leave me here. Get away. Just leave me here!"

Like before, I aimed my competitive arrogance at the people I was around the most. It didn't take long either. I checked into the unit knowing that I was better the minute I shook hands with the only other junior enlisted guy in the Intel shop: Corporal Butt Plug. At least, that's what I heard him say.

We were both corporals, and although he was senior to me (had been in longer), Butt Plug had never deployed and had never been overseas—he wasn't salty like me. He got all the bad DNA, with his short, squatty legs that didn't like to run; his gut and spare tire that showed through his shirt (big for Marine standards); his pudgy face and Dom DeLuise pencil-thin mustache; and his wrinkled uniform and boots that looked like they were polished with a Hershey Bar. *Hey, do you know Doofus?*

I thought Butt Plug was a lazy malingerer, and I couldn't let myself like him. I took more pride (deadly sin kind) in myself and my appearance. My boots were spit-shined, my uniforms were starched, and even my cover (hat) had crisp creases. I was tall, blond, in shape, and looked like a recruiting poster. I knew I did, for my new boss told me so.

"Hey, Marine! Where'd they find you—off of a poster or something?"

Gunny (short for gunnery sergeant; senior enlisted guy; my boss) was the one guy I didn't judge that year. For some reason, Gunny took a liking to me from the start. He reminded me of Louie (my old security guard boss). He showed an interest in me and seemed to respect my goals. And I respected him. He had been everywhere and done everything, so I begged him to send me to the grunts immediately—to *trade* me away if he could.

Gunny laughed in my face when I begged him, but he felt my passionate plea. "Give me a year, Audie. I'll train you more than anyone ever will. Do what I say and I'll get you to the grunts." I liked what I heard but had to correct him about my name. "No, devil dog. You remind me of Audie Murphy. Look him up one day, son. You might learn something."

Whatever, Gunny. I don't watch old war movies.

Gunny kept his word. He sent me to every training exercise and to every advanced training school he could possibly find. I was on the rifle range four times that year, and I became an expert shooter. I learned to drive a Humvee (highly mobile multi-wheeled vehicle) and scale mountains like a billy goat. Gunny had me in the desert three different times, each for thirty-day stints, to cross-train with the grunts—sleeping in the sand and learning groundside intelligence, map reading, and forward observation.

He even sent me with another unit to the United States-Mexico border. I rode around in a van with a border patrol agent every night for a month, drinking bad coffee and setting nonlethal ambushes for unsuspecting border crossers. Butt Plug didn't do any of this.

My favorite, though, was the individual training Gunny sent me to. One of the courses was in Bridgeport, California, for a two-week mountain survival course—like *Man Vs. Wild* before Bear Grylls made it a TV show. They dumped me in the high mountains of California to live on the land for eight days without any gear. It was a great test. I loved the training, even though I had to avoid hungry bears. The risks didn't matter to me. I was too busy stalking a young mountain lion like Elmer Fudd before I realized that I wasn't *that* hungry. *Hey, guy. You know that you actually do get to go home at some point, right?* I didn't care, and I took everything seriously. Even the many traps I set for unsuspecting squirrels, which by the way were much craftier than drunk, tired Marines trying to avoid ketchup and mustard packets.

But just as Thailand had propelled my thinking to another status in my immediate circle of douche bags, graduating SERE School put me in another class of Marines. SERE stands for Survival, Escape, Resistance, and Evasion. It's reserved for pilots, elite reconnaissance operators like Navy SEALS, Marine Force Recon, intelligence officers, and guys like me. It was the real deal when it came to learning how to survive in a prisoner of war (POW) situation and was by far the most intense and realistic training evolution I had ever experienced.

SERE was simply about life in captivity. To these people, life in captivity meant sneaking through the mountainous woods eating twigs, berries, and rabbits while navigating with a map during the day and at night from checkpoint to checkpoint to avoid capture by the enemy. Once captured, we learned to safely resist and survive life-threatening interrogations. The training area was tucked away deep inside the interior mountains outside San Diego, California—the kind of place where machine gun fire and bloodcurdling screams could easily be ignored. Surrounded by free-roam terrain, the prison camp looked just like the ones featured in the Chuck Norris/*Missing in Action* or Sly Stallone/*Rambo* movies. They kept us in individual "houses"—concrete boxes about the size of a washing machine, complete with coffee can toilets. The camp was complete with tall fences, a few guard towers, and loud speakers that pumped anti-American propaganda in bad soviet accents: *Amerikanskis is v-eak! Your country has forgotten you! Root in slop like pigs you are!*

SERE was military training, so they couldn't actually torture and kill you. They could, however, make you physically and severely uncomfortable with hard slaps to the face; repeated slams against aluminum walls; stress positions like prolonged crouching and stuffing; food, sleep, and light deprivation; cold temperatures; and water boarding (simulated drowning that makes you believe you will die). They also liked to shame you with nudity and play mental games that would haunt your soul. They wanted to break you or build you mentally, depending on how you looked at it.

Unbelievably, I thought I was most special when I was picked on. As one of the only Marines and one of the few enlisted to be in the course, I guess I stood out against the other guys. The Soviet-sounding guards (military trainers) locked on me the minute they rounded us up in the woods. Sitting in the back of a truck with a black hood over my face, I could hear them talk about me. "Look at him. He possess yellow hair. I never see yellow hair before. I make him purr like cat." (I suppose they don't have blond people in fake Russia . . . and maybe they sound a little like Tonto.)

All of our names were stripped once we got into the camp. Instead, we were called war criminals, and we were given numbers. I was war criminal #42, but the guards let me keep a name. They preferred to address me as "Yellow Hair" and make some sort of example or teaching aid out of me.

"Come to here, Yellow Hair. You have appeal of booger snot. Lepers avoid you. You are worthless and smell like goat testes."

"Come to here, Yellow Hair. You discharge more stupid than baby chicken."

"Come to here, Yellow Hair. Your commander is imbecile. Strip your clothes naked."

This was my least favorite. Not because I minded modeling my birthday suit in front my fellow war criminals. No. Because this usually happened at 2 a.m., and I didn't necessarily appreciate the fake Russian guards making me extend my arms out to my sides (like Jesus on the cross) and turn clockwise in place while they sprayed every inch of my bare skin with icy water from a garden hose. *Can you say shrinkage?*

93

"Yellow Hair, you have such tiny manhood. There is no way you can satisfy woman. You are homosexual, no?" Funny—my manhood was the last thing on my mind as I tried to spin perfect circles, trying not to get dizzy, and not let them break me.

"My, my, Yellow Hair, you have large anus. You are homosexual, no?" This one did make me laugh (on the inside). How ironic! *They directed me* to stand naked in the hills of Southern California, in the dark night, surrounded by grown men under the guise of "training," and somehow I was the homosexual. *Ironic . . . gently funny.*

Everybody suffered in that training, and I binged on it. I found the physical aspect of the training challenging, but it was manageable. I was Tuna Breath, for crying out loud. I had more sacrifice and discipline than a jackass mule, remember? The mental part was also a challenge, but I felt that I excelled. I couldn't be broken. I could make myself suffer more than any amount of pain someone could impose on me. I embraced all the training and I thought I performed well under pressure. I took their pain; I took their mind games; I kept my presence; I kept my life; I kept my secrets. I had traveled far beyond hiding my new identify from people like Coach Kent or keeping my obesity shame a secret. I could still be anybody I wanted to be. I truly believed that, and I could beat anyone—especially some dickhead navy trainer who sprayed me with cold water, naked in the middle of the night.

Gunny kept his word, and he trained me. He got me years of training in eleven months. It was common for me to return to the Cannon Cockers after being at a course, dump my gear in the barracks, and just look around. I started to look down on what I thought was mediocrity. I didn't make a single friend with the Cannon Cockers, mainly because I was always going somewhere. But I didn't try either, and it didn't really matter to me. I felt better than most guys because of all the training I was getting. I was doing things that I assumed many of them wouldn't even volunteer for, especially lazy people like Butt Plug.

When the grunts were kept away from me, I reacted with arrogance. I was striving to be the best; striving to be perfect; still trying to fulfill my need for certainty and significance in my life. I didn't realize it at the time, but most people don't strive to be perfect. I let myself become more ignorant to other aspects of life around me. I was still striving for something I didn't have, still bingeing on emotions. Me of all people, the former fat kid coming from my own place of weakness and fear, had become arrogant and judgmental. I beat my demon, and in doing so, I became one. I believed that made me special, better than everyone. *Man, you just can't kill me . . . Break glass in case of war.*

I didn't have any compassion for anyone I perceived as weak—none. I was alone and rigid—a silent competitor and an automaton. I stopped listening to my surroundings and learning from all people. I was Oscar the Grouch and a hermit by the ripe old age of twenty-two—well trained, surrounded by everyone, but deeply alone. I was still striving and still bingeing. I hated certain people deeply, and I forgot where I came from. I was lost and ignored my own flaws. Where in life did all that arrogance get me? If nothing else, it got me to the grunts. *Come to here, Yellow Hair!*

CHAPTER 8

MISERY LOVES ARROGANCE

Part of every misery is, so to speak, the misery's shadow or reflection: the fact that you don't merely suffer but have to keep on thinking about the fact that you suffer. I not only live each endless day in grief, but live each day thinking about living each day in grief.

—C. S. Lewis

How open are you about your true feelings? It may seem trivial but look at the act of greeting someone, for example. Do you tell people how you're really feeling? You know, when a friend, stranger, family member, or coworker asks, "How are ya?" or "What's up?"

As a kid in Burbank, "What's up?" was the common greeting. You had "What's up, bro?" and "What's up, dude?" and "What's up, man?" And with Disney Studios at the edge of town, we also had "What's up, Doc?" This was virtually the same thing as "How are ya?" Who knew if people were really interested in hearing what was really up or how you really were? But the casual, acceptable response, no matter how you felt, was always "Not much, man!" No one (especially guys) ever said "I'm unsatisfied today," "I'm anxious today," "I'm lonely today," or "You're fucking pissing me off!"

I suppose this is an ordinary scenario for many people in everyday life. It certainly was for me once I burrowed into the Marines. Even if I felt this way, saying "You're fucking pissing me off!" would have never passed as a standard greeting, especially to anyone with authority. In the Marines, when asked how you were doing, the proper reply, the standard response, was always "Outstanding!" It didn't matter if your feet were blistered and your crotch was raw from all the hikes. When asked how you were by a superior, "Outstanding, sir!" was the expected reply. Same thing if you were tired and hungry: "Outstanding, sir!" If you were lonely, pissed, happy, or sad, "Outstanding, sir!" was never the wrong answer.

Outstanding, sir! was simply part of Marine vocabulary for me. Just like "cover" (hat), "rack" (bed), and "field day" (cleanup). The fact is that we were trained to respond this way beginning on the first day of boot camp. Maybe it was about not showing weakness or vulnerability. Perhaps this positive affirmation promoted motivation and improved morale on some level. Either way, I never thought too long and hard about it. I thought I was "outstanding" all the time so why not say it? I was motivated, having drunk the Kool-Aid and swallowed the red pill of truth. So what if we had to do many things that sucked? The common thought among my brand of Marines: "Marines aren't happy if they aren't bitching, and I'm the happiest motherfucker here." *Outstanding!*

Looking back, I know that Marine officers weren't always looking for this reply. I'm sure they wanted and needed to hear more. As leaders, their responsibility stretched way deeper than what my young arrogant mind was willing to acknowledge at twenty-three years old. But if you looked up "marine officer" online you might find something like this:

The Marine Corps Officer is a leader, a warrior and an upstanding citizen instilled with the special trust and confidence of our nation to lead its expeditionary force.

Distinguished by a Commission

Officers are college graduates who have earned and accepted an appointment by the President of the United States. Their commission gives them the responsibility of leading Marines as they defend the Constitution of the United States.

Doug Pedersen

Trained by Leaders to Be Leaders

During initial training, Marine Officers learn from experienced senior officers. Then, specialized training instructors will help them refine skills in their specific field. This process ensures that new officers can lead from the front.
(Taken from http://web.usf.edu/nrotc/nrotc/Marine-Corps-Careers.htm)

So by their very definition, officers were upstanding, distinguished, college-educated, responsible leaders from the front. If you looked up "enlisted man" (which is what I was), you would find:

A serviceman who ranks below a commissioned officer.
(Taken from http://www.thefreedictionary.com/serviceman)
Or, how we commonly thought of ourselves, *someone who works for a living!*

In the end, we were taught in boot camp that officers were the leaders, the deciders, the commanders. They did the thinking. We, the enlisted guys, did the work. Officers were educated. They were the lieutenants, captains, majors, colonels, and generals. Officers were gentlemen, managers, and military executives. But if you asked me back in the first few years of my enlistment, Marine officers were like Greek gods or maybe unicorns: you rarely saw one of them up close, if at all. And if you did, even though you didn't know what they did all day, you knew that they were rare and you didn't want them involved in your day-to-day business.

My opinion of officers changed once I finally was stationed with the grunts. Luckily, I was sent to an infantry battalion in California. A good buddy from MCT and Intel school was already stationed there (Greg, or Greggor, as I referred to him). We were good friends and would now work together. This was also the same unit where I (we) reunited with Sergeant Sanchez. It wasn't hard to fit in, and I loved it. *Good night, motherfucker!*

As an Intel guy, I lived and worked with the scout sniper platoon. This group consisted of twelve to fifteen highly trained special grunts. Snipers were the best of the best in the unit, the guys who could survive in the jungle on their own, deep behind enemy lines. They were the ones who

98

would lie on their stomachs in a tall grass field for three days, stalking closer to a target for a chance at that perfect shot. Vietnam-era snipers like Carlos Hathcock established this mystical reputation by racking up more than fifty confirmed kills from a single hilltop. I wasn't a sniper by any stretch, but they did accept me as one of their own, and we were close. We tasked them; they dispatched targets.

Not all our days were spent on patrols, rappel towers, rifle ranges, or in some sort of exotic training. There were many instances where I was in the battalion headquarters (HQ). HQ was located at Camp San Mateo, a smaller camp on the larger base, just over the hill from where I attended Marine Combat Training (MCT) under Sergeant Sanchez. The aged but well-kept two-story administration building sat inches away from golden brown hills, trails, and the Southern California coastline. It was also the place where the battalion commander (colonel) sat to make all the rules for the seven hundred or so Marines under his command (our snipers included). All of his officers had offices, including the Intel officer who happened to be my boss.

The intelligence office was on the second floor—smack dab in the middle of the building. It might remind you of the office that adjunct professors share at a community college or the PE teacher's office in the back of the gym. Fit for one adult man, the only open space in this office was a four-by-four-foot patch of carpet immediately inside the front door. If you stood there and surveyed the room, to the immediate left sat a card table-sized surface where the DOS computer and dot matrix printer sat. Two gray government desks sat side by side, facing the door. Nothing but phones and loose paper occupied these surfaces. A four-shelf bookcase sat behind each desk, which contained faded Marine publications and training manuals. Split between the desks, on top of one of the shelves, sat a Zenith television set straight out of the 1970s. A brown pleather two-seat couch was placed to the right of the carpet patch and completed the clockwise scan of the office. Movie poster-sized maps of the base hung on the wall, and although everything was aged like old French cheese, the office was spotless. Naturally, this was where our lieutenant hung out most of the time.

Our lieutenant looked nothing like a Greek god or a mystical unicorn. He was maybe twenty-eight years old at the time; his hair was Marine short and graying on the sides. He wasn't Jimmy Two Times, but he did repeat words in his sentences, in his sentences. He laughed like a chipmunk, like a chipmunk, and had a nervous energy that kept him from sitting in his chair or listening to other people, other people. We all wore camouflage uniforms, but after a few incidents like my "check-in moment," I couldn't help but wonder what on earth he was doing in the Marine Corps. Mainly because he was the only Marine I ever heard talk about the stock market.

I remember walking in to officially check in and meet him for the first time. He was standing up and bent over the Zenith, trying to adjust a flimsy set of rabbit ears.

"Corporal Pedersen reporting as ordered, sir!" I stood at attention on the carpet.

"At ease. At ease. Do you know how to crush a man's windpipe with a short punch?"

I noticed his northeastern accent. "Excuse me, sir?"

"Here—stand here right." He pointed at the only open spot in the tightly packed office. I didn't need to move an inch, as I was already standing there.

I looked around, and one of the salty snipers whom I hadn't met was sitting on the brown pleather couch and shaking his head, looking skeptical. "You can't do it, sir. I keep telling you that you need more of a windup."

Sitting at the computer table, Greggor felt inclined to interject: "Sir, can this wait? I'm sure he can do it. But we need to finish this report for the S-3. Hey, Pedersen—what's up?"

The lieutenant abandoned the Zenith and stepped from behind his desk to the open spot on the floor. He squared up in front of me and placed both his hands on my shoulders, like a loose Greco-Roman clinch. "This is what you do . . . what you do, right. Straighten your arm and place the tip of your middle finger at the target."

He removed his right hand from my shoulder and straightened his arm until his middle finger touched the center of my chest. "Let the force run from your butt cheeks to your arm . . . from your butt cheeks, right, then make a fist and strike." He made a fist and punched my chest with the force of a five-year-old.

Ugh! "Nice one, sir?" I glanced at the guys with my *Is he serious* look, wondering if I was supposed to act as if it hurt.

"I didn't want to crush your chest for real. But you get the idea, right." The Lieutenant chuckled like a chipmunk.

"I told you—you need more of a windup, sir. A strike like that wouldn't even tickle your sorority sister." The salty sniper chuckled. "Hey, Pedersen, what's up? Welcome to scout snipers."

"Sir, the S-3? He's waiting," Greggor said.

"Corporal Pedersen, Corporal Pedersen, do you know how to work rabbit ears?" The lieutenant stepped back to the Zenith and tugged at the makeshift antennae as if they were leftover tent poles.

He fiddled with the ears for a few more seconds. "Corporal Pedersen, Corporal Pedersen, what time is it?"

"Thirteen hundred, sir. Why?" It was one o'clock in the afternoon military time.

"Why? It's time for the lieutenant's run, right. See if you can fix this thing and tell me what MS is doing." He snatched a small gym bag from behind his desk and scooted out of the office like a guy who just farted in the elevator.

"MS? What the fuck is that?" I inquired to the other boys.

"It's stock broker shit. The symbol for Microsoft, I think. He's trying to make his fortune. But don't worry, Pedersen. Take a seat; he'll be back and forget all about it," Greggor explained, motioning to the extra desk next to the lieutenants.

"Microsoft? What the fuck is that?" I inquired again. It was 1996, almost 1997, and I had no knowledge of such *mystical* things.

Scenes like this played out many times over the next three months. If I wasn't out with the snipers, I sat at one of the extra desks while Greggor worked the computer (I didn't know how to use it). We discussed training, debated tactics, and planned operations until Scooter (my private name for the lieutenant) got bored and wanted to show off his aikido. I suppose that's all we could do together. I didn't understand the stock market and had no idea who Dow Jones was. So as the new guy, I was his training dummy and the guy he used to demonstrate how to *katate dori* (break an arm), *ushiro kubishime* (choke a throat), *tantōtori* (block a knife strike), and *kickapecka* (take a kick to the Jimmy). There was always some new lame move with him. "Corporal Pedersen, Corporal Pedersen, do you know how to do a *tachitori*?" How could I break his prep school heart and tell him "Yes, sir, I know the 'sword takeaway'?" *Whatever* . . .

Despite his quirks, it was natural for me to accept him, as I had been trained as an officer, and I thought that as a grunt officer, he should be better than I was in every way. He was the leader, the one who had been trained to do so. By the Marine's definition, he was upstanding, distinguished, and college educated, a leader from the front. I was an enlisted man and below him, so I needed to listen. In theory, he was in command. That is what I believed at the time.

It was difficult to keep Scooter on a pedestal after our first extensive field training evolution together. This was my chance to see the theory of his leadership style play out in an environment away from his cozy office—in the raw elements . . . in the field.

Several months after I checked in, our entire unit was sent to the Mountain Warfare Training Center—also known as Pickel Meadows—in Bridgeport, California. Sure, it sounded like the kind of place Yogi and Boo-boo Bear might have a picnic, but the Marines got there first and made it a training area. In reality, the forest was dense and the herd of mountain peaks darted upward, way above the warm air at sea level. The valleys were deep, and there wasn't any flat ground anywhere. It was the kind of place from which you could touch the clouds. It was wintertime, and the temperatures dipped below thirty degrees on a daily basis. Pristine snow blanketed the jagged ground, and the tall pine trees like a massive white comforter. It wasn't Everest, but your calves, back, and lungs wouldn't know the difference.

The training was meant to simulate the rigid and rugged mountain environment in North Korea—like if we ever had to go there and fight. This was also the place where we were going to learn how to cross-country and Telemark ski, snowshoe, and do many patrols and mountain warfare training exercises. Everyone carried at least eighty pounds of gear, trudging through the snow every day like wooly mammoths goats, going from one training evolution to the other. We slept in four-man collapsible tents and pretty much lived on top of each other to stay warm. Each night, however, the tent needed to be buried in the snow to protect us from the harsh elements and to hide our position. It was hard physical work after a long, physical day, digging with kid-sized shovels like junior archeologists. We were snow nomads, and Greggor and I had the unfortunate pleasure of sharing a tent with Scooter for the entire month.

Lucky for me, I knew Bridgeport well. These mountains were the same ones I lived in during a mountain survival course the year before—alone instead of with a unit. (Remember the *Man Vs. Wild*, Bear Gryls reference?) Having been there, I was familiar with the territory, and I knew a lot about the environment. I knew which twigs and berries to eat, although there wasn't much in the wintertime, and I knew that the rivers and streams contained *Giardia*—a single-celled parasite that can cause gastrointestinal illness. Giardia was like a bad breakup, nasty and could make you lose sleep for weeks. So you had to be careful with what you drank, either purifying everything with iodine pills or preferably by boiling it in a fire. If you didn't, you were bound to get violently ill, with intense diarrhea, stomach cramps, bloating, gas, and fatigue. These symptoms could cause serious damage in a real survival situation. Of course, the trainers went over all of this stuff again, and you were fine if you listened.

Scooter certainly didn't listen. Instead, he "cocooned" several hours after our first hike up deep into the mountains. *Cocooning* was the word that the trainers used for someone who shut down because of the cold, rejecting it altogether, literally cocooning in his clothes (layer upon layer; hands in pockets; chin on chest; knees locked together; alone, quiet, and still).

So what if he was cold? All of us were cold. On the first night, instead of helping Greggor and me dig the hole for our tent, Scooter put on every piece of cold weather snow clothing he could find and sat on a fallen pine tree. He pulled his hood over his face and tugged the drawstring until only a small breathing hole was exposed to the frigid air—he had it over his eyes and everything. He sat there by himself while the whole unit—his snipers, Greggor, and me, and even other officers scattered across the narrow valley—worked to make camp for the night. He couldn't see that work would actually keep his body warm, even though he was exhausted and cold. Instead, the cold log reached into his anus like a pickpocket and stole his core temperature. He did all the wrong things to deal with the rigors of the environment; he cocooned early and often.

"Sir, why don't you get your e-tool and help us dig? It will warm you up," Greggor said while heaving snow like a garbage man on overtime.

From his spot on the wet log through his hood hole, he ignored Greggor and said, "Corporal Pedersen, Corporal Pedersen, what time is it?" I told him that it was five thirty, and before I finished heaving my snow scoop, he said, "Corporals, I need to talk to the company commander about tomorrow's training schedule. We're snowshoeing, right. Keep digging. I'll be back to help finish it out."

Greggor snapped at him. "The company commander is digging his own hole! Why don't . . ." But Scooter had already hopped off the log and scooted off into the woods. I bit my tongue and kept working.

Scooter never came back to "finish it out." When he did return, Greggor and I were done digging. The tent was up, and we had rolled out our gear for the night. The hole was four or five feet deep and big enough to fit a Volkswagen. We were sweaty, and I was bitter.

Scooter returned just as we finished working. "Nice job, men. Set my sleeping bag up while you're at it. Put mine in the middle of you two, right. I need to keep an eye on you." And he trudged off in the snow again, this time in the other direction.

When Scooter came back, we had the stove going. We could see that he was freezing and had probably been sitting (cocooned) somewhere by himself. I handed him a cup of hot chocolate from our rations and tried to explain why he needed to do physical work—how it wasn't beneath him. Work was actually a survival technique and necessary. But he wasn't interested or listening; he was too cold and too proud.

"Corporal Pedersen, Corporal Pedersen," he interrupted. "What time is it? I wonder what the market closed at today."

Whatever . . .

This routine continued day after day. I took note of his unwillingness to do anything tough, and the chip on my shoulder was back. In my mind, he was an officer and was supposed to be a leader—"from the front." So it was hard for me not to wonder, *How can this guy lead me when he's such a pussy?* He never lifted a finger when we had to bury the tent at night. Sure, Greggor and I were cold and hungry, and he always managed to disappear, even when other officers were burying their tents. They led from the front as they were supposed to. Why couldn't Scooter? I got so annoyed that I completely stopped talking to him. But for some reason, he latched on to me like a scared child, always tugging on my shirttails and asking me what time it was every ten minutes, as if he were my child and I was responsible for telling him when to eat, when to sleep, when to train, and what was next. "Corporal Pedersen, what time is it? Corporal, Pedersen, what time is it? Is it time to eat?"

Fuck off, sir! Where's your watch?

Digging the hole for our house was hard work. But the worst job of all was lighting the single-flame propane stove in the morning. It was wretched because whoever drew this task had to leave the warm safety of his sleeping bag to do it. Considering the fact that we slept in the nude, greeting Mother Nature in subfreezing temperatures to light the stove was an admirable sacrifice for the other guys in the tent. Of course, Greggor and I (and every other Marine) thought it was most fair to take turns. The other grunt officers did this too. They participated. With three men in the tent, it followed that one would only have to do this evil job every third day. But Scooter managed to squeak out of this one too. He bribed us at first: "I'll give you all five's on your proficiency report if you take my turn." After a few days, he used his rank: "Light the stove. That's an order, right." After a few days more, he didn't even respond.

"Sir? Sir?" Silence. *Whatever.*

To get back at him, Greggor and I planned a snowball ambush. It was a great caper because we thought it was best to attack him when he least expected it—and when he was most vulnerable. So after the first week in the snow while digging the hole (again), Greggor and I waited for Scooter's daily excuse.

"Corporal Pedersen, Corporal Pedersen, what time is it?" When I told him it was five thirty in the afternoon, he announced, "Set up the tent here, put my bag in the middle, and start the stove. I'm going to take a *shit-towski.* Toss me my day pack."

My part of the hole was already knee deep; his orders were always late and useless. I reached across to his gear and snuck the toilet paper out of it before tossing it to him. *Go ahead and wipe with the snow, or a leaf, or a rabbit, numbnuts.*

After he trudged off, Greggor and I rounded up four of our sniper buddies from the next hole over and patrolled back behind the poop tree that Scooter had selected in the distance. We hid behind a large fallen pine, about fifteen feet up the snowy hill from where Scooter sat on the bucket. We each worked with care to make a stack of wet snowballs and took our positions in a line behind the tree. With our green ski masks pulled over our faces, we leaped up and launched the first barrage, ducking immediately after throwing them. Scooter got pelted like a car in a hailstorm. *Splat!*

"Hey! What's that?" He was half smiling, partially confused at first. Maybe he thought it was other officers playing a prank on him. *College boys.*

We stood up again and launched another round. *Splat, splat, splat!* The snowballs found their mark.

He stood up from the bucket, pants down. "Stop it, Marines! Who are you? Reveal your faces. I'm an officer!" His commands became more irritated.

Who talks like that? I laughed.

Another barrage followed. *Splash, mash, dash!*

"What the fuck! I'm going to . . ." We interrupted him with another volley. *Boom, bang, bing!* He was pissed off, but he couldn't abandon his spot on the throne to chase us. *Ancient Chinaman say, "Never run with poopy butt unless you want dirty feet!"*

We retreated to our holes to catch our breath and laugh at our leader. Our celebration lasted only a few minutes because we didn't want him to know it was us, although a two-year-old could have figured this one out. But Scooter didn't come through the tree line for at least twenty or thirty minutes. Who knew what he was doing all that time, but he had no idea it was us. He didn't even mention it.

"What's the poop, sir? There's nothing like building a sturdy cabin in the fresh snow, eh?" I chided. He didn't get it.

Instead of ranting about the snowballs, he surprised us with this next declaration: "Corporal Pedersen., Corporal Pedersen, do you have any TP? I'm out . . ."

Before he could finish his thought, Greggor interrupted him. "You didn't wipe, sir? You need to wash your ass before coming in here." He motioned to the buried tent.

"Yeah, you need to wash your ass, sir!" I reinforced.

Scooter's eyes glazed. "I could do it in the river, right. That would be a good picture too!"

"You won't do it. It's freezing in there. Besides, it's just a stream. You don't have the guts." Greggor continued to goad him.

"Bad idea, sir. Go back to the bucket and use your canteen. It . . ." But Scooter wasn't listening to me.

"Corporal Pedersen, Corporal Pedersen, is the stove on? I'll jump in and jump right out. Take a picture; I want my friends to see." And he trudged over to the stream.

So he wanted to pose like a tough guy and wash his ass in the river. Not a photo I'd like to share with my family, but then again, I wasn't Scooter. I thought it was odd, too, that he chose this option—although he was always more about appearances than truths. To my shock, the fool actually stripped off all of his clothes and sat in the shallow stream, naked as a newborn baby. I remember thinking how stupid that was: for starters, you would never willingly expose yourself in icy water in a survival situation. That's a good way to get hypothermia, especially if you didn't know how to start a fire and warm yourself, which he didn't. Also, the water was full of bacteria and disease, and you didn't need to drink the water to contract *Giardia*. It could seep into other openings like your nose, eyes, and in this case, his unsuspecting butthole. But Scooter never listened. He jumped in the stream, sitting on the bottom of the cold, slimy rock bed, hiding his privates with both hands as I stood on the bank snapping pictures on his disposable camera like a paparazzi. "Good one, sir!" *Smile, ass wipe!*

Forgetting about the river bath, my anger at Scooter grew deeper a few days later. Again, he refused to take his turn lighting the stove in the freezing morning air. I was at my wit's end. I was furious at him but didn't say anything. I rooted around in the tent like a pouty kid, but I bit my tongue. I didn't know what passive aggressive meant back then, but Greggor and I finally decided to make Scooter earn his comfort. So we didn't warm the tent that morning for the lieutenant. Instead, we bared our bodies to the cold, got dressed in the tent, and lit the stove outside. We made coffee and oatmeal and warmed up on the snow porch we'd dug the night before.

"Corporal Pedersen, Corporal Pedersen, what time is it?" he yelled from his sleeping bag. "How long before formation?" He wanted to stay inside the warm sleeping bag as long as he could.

"What time, what time, what time." I was so pissed off and frustrated with him. I flipped him off through the tent. I mimicked his faces and voices to Greggor. I grabbed my crotch and motioned for him to suck it. And then we turned off the stove and got really quiet.

"Corporal Pedersen, Corporal Pedersen. Is the stove still lit? Bring it in here." Greggor and I responded with silence. His pleas for warmth increased, but Greggor and I just sat there on our packs, nice and warm, watching the snowdrifts. We required Scooter to feel the cold air on his naked body that day, which was the beginning of his end.

As Greggor and I snickered to each other, I finally heard the zipper from the tent open. It was Scooter; his hands were shaking, and his lips were pursed but not quite blue. At least he was dressed. He looked like a frozen junkie hunting for another hit as he asked, "Corporal Pedersen, what time is it? What are you guys doing? The stove is easy, right. Toss me your lighter."

Scooter located the stove that sat on the snow wall on the edge of our hole. He jacked the tiny pencil-sized pump in and out like a humping Chihuahua. He pumped so hard and so fast that the propane gas leaked out of the top seal, onto the tank, and onto his hands. He couldn't even tell. The air was so cold and the propane was so light; he couldn't feel the gas on his frozen skin. Scooter was more than numb and in a hurry; he didn't notice that he had over-pressurized the stove and turned himself into a potential human blowtorch.

Still, I tossed him my bad lighter and looked at Greggor. There was a little concern that he would blow himself up, but I bet that he wouldn't be able to get the goddamned thing lit anyway. He needed matches in this weather. I just wanted to see if he would try to. *What an idiot!* He flicked the flint with his swollen gassy hands, but the cold air had robbed his dexterity. Even so, I moved my seat across the snow hole to the opposite snow wall just in case he ignited the stove and set himself on fire. *Oh well,* I thought. *It's survival of the fittest out here!* He never flinched or showed concern. He flicked the lighter ten or twenty times. Greggor and I just left him there with his gas, his broken lighter, and his frozen self.

I couldn't help but remember thinking how much he'd talked himself up back on the base. In the rear, he bragged like a teenage boy around a group of young virgins. A lot of good his aikido or famous Boston school did him now. Now we were in the field, in God's country, cold, wet, and expected to fight. Instead, he collapsed. He couldn't function, and I saw him as a liability, never as a leader of Marines and definitely not as somebody that I could respect or follow. How could I follow him? He was a cocooner; I was a poster boy that bought into the invincible image that Marine officers were supposed to have. I was tough, the best, perfect, and could do anything that anyone could throw at me. I could never let myself respect him as a Marine or as an officer after that. I just couldn't. I was more than let down.

Despite losing total respect for him, deep down I didn't want him dead. That night after a long day of snowshoeing around, Greggor and I took pity on Scooter. He had been quiet all day and said even less when it was time to dig the hole and set the tent. We dug it and set up his gear in the middle. I despised doing so, but there was no way he would've made it through the night without possibly getting ill. I kept telling myself, *Just dig the fucking hole. At least he can still walk on his own. You don't want to carry him next, do you?* We finished the hole and went to sleep without saying good night.

Sometime during the freezing night, I heard the zipper of the tent's front flap open. *Zip!* Scooter was wrestling around a lot, but what else was new? Greggor snored like a lumberjack on the other side of the tent, but I stayed quiet just to see what Scooter was up to. Apparently, he had been outside and was reentering our hooch.

"Corporal Pedersen! Corporal Pedersen! What time is it?" he said with a frantic whisper.

I couldn't believe this asshole was waking me up to ask what time it was—again! "It's one thirty in the morning, sir! We don't need to be up for another four hours. Go back to—"

Greggor still snored as Scooter interrupted me. "Be advised: I have *explosive* diarrhea, and there's blood in my stool. That's bad, right? I'm going to wake the doc and get evacuated."

No pun intended, I'm sure.

Scooter collected his gear from the center of the tent as if he had just won a large poker pot. I never saw him move that fast in the two and a half weeks that he was there. I couldn't see his face, but he must have looked relieved to get out of his snowy hell. I quietly smiled to myself as I lay cocooned in my warm sleeping bag. I'm sure he *did* in fact have explosive diarrhea, and I knew he suffered. I knew it was *Giardia* and his little naked stunt in the creek that now ailed him. By this time, Greggor had awakened, and when Scooter dismissed himself from the tent, we both said in unison, "Good night, sir!"

A few hours later Greggor and I woke up in the predawn hours. We basked in the peace of being rid of Scooter. It was as if a wart had been cut off my nose. We sipped coffee while watching the sunrise from our snow hole. Greggor and I laughed and mimicked Scooter's voice: *"I have explosive diarrhea, right!"* After a few more jeers, we noticed where Scooter had been most of the night. It was like a crime scene—or in this case, a *crap* scene. We followed his footprints that disturbed the smooth snow pack, leading up a small hill to a big tree. It looked as if he had been up there, probably crouched at the knees for hours, exploding away. It was a mess, and he'd even left his green undershorts up there in the trampled brown snow. *Oh, God! Wet fart!*

I shook my head, so glad to have him gone and away from me. "Scoots" deserved worse. I didn't care a bit how sick he was or even if he was going to be okay. Scoots was incompetent in this environment; he was dead weight . . . a liability. It was even worse when we finished everything and were back at the base a few weeks later. How could I respect him after that? I saw him as a fake, and I couldn't stand to listen to or be around him. We were always first; he was always last. He led from his cocoon, and I let these little things build up like the Great Wall of China. I let him make me miserable.

Unfortunately for my Marine binge, Scoots wasn't the only officer that I let betray me. In the three years that followed, I served with two other officers who were also fakes, just like Scoots. Another couldn't make decisions or stand up for his troops—he was a yes man. And still another who wanted nothing more than to get out of the Marine Corps and hunt deer all day; he was lazy, hated work, and cheated on his wife—so much for integrity. One officer was eager to lead, but he was a tattletale. And then there was Scoots—he led the way for my misery and disappointment to grow toward these weak leaders. What gave these guys the right to lead me? But who was I to be so righteous?

I loved the grunts, and despite my arrogance and my misery, I loved the entire Marine Corps. This was my love affair, my validation, my identity. I binged on it, and I was committed to the life with 100 percent of my body and soul, even though I allowed a metric ton of negativity into the experience. But somehow my bingeing nature and arrogant stance made it okay for me to get very irritated (and angry) with my leaders and the officers in charge of me. I was more than pissed off, and I couldn't get past my disappointment. I was resentful and carried this misery around every time I saw one of them. I couldn't take what I thought was their bad decisions, their lack of leadership, and their hypocrisy anymore. I let them get deep into my soul, and I let myself get angry, unhappy, and miserable.

Somewhere along the way, I started to focus on problems that I couldn't control. I blamed *them;* I judged *them*; I let *them* make me unhappy. Somewhere along the way, I developed a long memory and never let anything go. Looking back, when asked, "What's up?" by a superior, I held my misery deep inside myself, bottled up like a cheap wine, when perhaps I should have been brutally honest and said, "You're fucking pissing me off!" instead of "Outstanding, sir!"

CHAPTER 9

BLACK PANTHER PARTY

A dream doesn't become reality through magic; it takes sweat, determination, and hard work.

—Colin Powell

The cuddly cat, as evil as it was, had peaceful eyes. I suppose that's what drew me in the most. He appeared on the coffee table like a magic trick (*poof!*). Or like a panther that leaped from its perch in a high tree. His whip like tail stood straight in the air as he sauntered toward my spot on the couch. His bright yellow eyes were wide open; his ears were pinned back by harmless curiosity; and he greeted me with a soft kitty hello: *Meow-purr.*

I couldn't help but reach my hand out to pet the evil cat's thick black fur. Despite my arrogance at the time, deep within my core, I was still a giver, a lover, a natural pleaser, so I found it very easy to pet him. Besides, I had nothing else to do. The cat's owner, my new friend, was nowhere to be found. Our friendship was vague, but we seemed familiar enough for the guy to leave me alone in his living room while he grabbed us beers, or checked his mail, or took a dump.

Also a sucker for affection, the evil cat's purr filled the room as I pet him. He must have felt comforted too, as he surrendered his neck to my petting. We were friends now. He turned his face to the sky so I could rub under his chin. After a long rubdown, the evil cat turned his head to the right, eyes shut with bliss, and gave me the back of his ears. His purrs grew louder and stronger like the steady roll of a snare drum. Then the evil cat slowly twisted his hind end around and maneuvered his body under my fingers to stroke his own back—from his neck to his tail. His haunches raised in delight. He trusted me like a brother by this point, and we were in love.

Hsssss! The cuddly cat jerked up. His pupils now dilated—the size of big black marbles.

Again: *Hsssss!* The cuddly cat swiped a free claw at me. He struck like a lightning bolt; one of his extended claws ripped the belly of my forearm open.

With a soft, nurturing voice I said, "Hey, easy, friend. It's okay. No more petting; no problem." I looked at the wound but didn't acknowledge the pain. The cut was deep, like a filleted fish. *Damn, man! No reason to panic.*

Hsssss! The cuddly cat's eyes glimmered and dilated larger. I should have known that more mischief was coming. He struck again with ferocious speed. This time he sliced my other forearm. Shocked, I still told myself, *It's only a scratch.* But this laceration went to the bone. "No need to panic, little guy. It's okay. I won't . . ."

Hsssss! Another quick swipe from his extended razors followed . . . and another . . . and another. Before I knew it, three of the cuddly cat's claws had sliced through my skin and were stuck deep inside my muscle tissue. I had no choice but to hold him now. We were attached. Sure, we were friends, brothers even, but this was like shaking hands with Freddy Krueger. The pain was too intense to ignore; I had to do something but didn't want to panic. *Fuck! What the fuck, cat!* Blood flowed from the gashes in my arm and spilled into a pool on the floor. The cuddly cat never lost his gaze. I could see his evil intentions, but I couldn't retaliate. I felt bad for the cuddly cat. I loved him and could only think, *You're just a cat—small, furry, and affectionate. Calm down, please!*

Hsssss! He swung his last free claw like an axe and buried it deep in my forearm. The pain shot to my brain like a .50-caliber bullet.

Ahhhhh! My heart raced with fear. This had to be my fault. I must have scared the evil cat. Did he feel cornered? Is he just defending himself? In disbelief, I tried to gently remove each claw from my skin and let him run away.

Hsssss! Before I could remove anything, the cuddly cat squirmed violently with rabid movement. It was like having a porcupine balled up in my hands. His claws ripped deeper into my skin. The pain throbbed through my limbs and felt like someone was cutting my fingers with scissors, ripping my fingernails out with pliers, and pounding nails into my palms all at the same time. *Ahhhhh! Why? Ahhhhh!*

Hsssss! Balled up in my hands, stuck like Velcro, his claws imbedded, welded, to my arms and hands and bones, I brought him close to my face. The blood dripped freely on my chest and lap. I was soaked in it, my heart broken. Razor-sharp cuts to the bone exposed my muscles and nerves. I had to ask him why.

"Judas! You betrayed me. We were doing so well. Why?" I screamed. He looked at me with innocence. His eyes turned back to yellow and appeared peaceful and helpless. I felt the bond we shared at first and thought, *It's okay, kitty. I forgive . . .*

Hsssss!

Fuck!

The cuddly cat struck again like a rattlesnake. His front canine teeth, sharp as razors, deep as nails, penetrated my cheek and chin. The pain rushed to my heart. *Beat-beat . . . beat-beat . . . beat-beat. What now?*

Rage finally boiled my blood. Reluctantly and regretfully, I maneuvered my hands near the cat's neck, inflicting more pain on myself with each reach. His jaws pulsated, inching his teeth deeper into my face.

Once at his neck, I squeezed with all my strength, with all my anger. I fought the pain and strangled the cuddly cat's neck. I let out another bloodcurdling cry. *Ahhhhh!* This time it was a war cry, and I slowly suffocated every breath out of the cuddly cat until he stopped moving. I was out of breath and maybe in shock. *What just happened? Thank God it's over.* I cried.

With the evil cat dead, I still needed to pluck his teeth and claws. I started with the teeth in my face. It was like unhooking a fish. I nearly passed out as the teeth ripped out of my skin, just as they had ripped in. I repeated the process with each of his now lifeless claws. One at a time. *Ahhhhh!* Tears of joy, of fear, of anger, and of relief flowed from my eyes—almost as freely as the blood that now covered the room. *Ahhhhh! Why? At least I'm free.*

The cat was limp and lifeless. He lay in my bloody hands like a fresh sacrifice. With disgust and relief, I launched the cat as hard as I could like a football into the other room. *Thud!* Maybe the dead cat hit the wall. Maybe he hit the coffee table. Maybe he hit my new buddy. Some friend he was. At least I was alive. What a Greek tragedy.

My heart skipped as I tried to process what had just happened. The pain was so intense. My skin was shredded and torn. The blood was slippery. I was soaked from head to toe. My arms quivered; my hands shook; my heart was broken in half. Then the pain rushed to my core: *Ahhhh! Why? At least I'm alive. At least I'm free. Why? Ahhhhh!*

*   *   *

You know there is a problem when you have a recurring dream like this. Even though I wasn't aware of its meaning at first, I couldn't ignore the physical responses my body had during these dreams. They were so intense and real. After waking up in horror, I would discover my hands and arms contorted under my body or pressed against my pillow or the wall, to the point where the circulation had stopped. Literally, my hands and arms were usually asleep, pulsating, with the pins and needles feeling that paralyzes you if you crouch too long or if you sit on the toilet too long. These painful sensations usually distracted me from noticing right away that I was also soaked in sweat and my heart was pounding like a jackhammer. As I said, whatever it meant, I didn't need NASA to tell me: "Houston, we have a problem!"

In reality, I knew that things weren't *right* with me on the inside. I could feel it, all of my negativity and bitterness. But at the time, I thought I was invincible, not vulnerable and sensitive. I believed that I was full grown at twenty-five years old and closing in on my stint with the Marines. I was a crusty sergeant, having been to over ten countries and lived overseas for half my time. The Marines awarded me achievement medals, good conduct medals, overseas service medals; I served with the grunts (and snipers), and I was a leader of young Marines by now. I had lived on ship, been south of the equator a few times and performed at a high level with everything I did. I had accomplished everything I'd set out to do in the Marine Corps—except actually fight a war.

No. My service was a peace placeholder in time (1994-2000). I was a defender of freedom who never needed to act, a young man still chasing significance and unable to see why I was miserable deep on the inside. I wasn't "outstanding." I was unhappy and bitter, and I never expressed any parts of my dark side. I just never acknowledged it and couldn't recognize it, nor could I tell anyone or express my true self. I truly didn't know how. Just like the oxymoronic attitude I kept as an obese binge-eating teenager. Nothing had changed with my emotional intelligence, and I was still very good at hiding my emotions and controlling the image I let people see of me while hiding my true feelings.

It took me eight months of reflection to figure this dream out. But in the end, on a random afternoon, sitting in my barracks room in Japan, I mentioned it to a buddy during a light conversation so we could laugh about it. I told him the dream in a humble, self-deprecating way. Once I got into the description, the dream's symbolism jumped right out at me. It was simple and clear: the cuddly/evil cat scenario represented the exact relationship (scenario) I kept with many people at the time. It was how I viewed and felt that I had to treat people in my life that had wronged me in some way, especially my direct peers and leaders (the people near me). The cat represented the people I grew to disregard, judge, hate, cut off, strangle. I took their faults personally, and over time, I eventually turned those people into my enemies—conflicted and regretfully so, until I had to "strangle" the relationship just to get away from the anger *they* caused *me*.

Cutting off the relationship usually meant that I stopped talking to them. I wouldn't ignore them, but I wouldn't engage them either. I would do my best to work around them and do everything myself. When I was alone, I would talk to myself. I would curse, or *motherfuck*, them in private. I paced in my room, replaying whatever it was they said or did that bothered me that day. Sometimes I threw things at the wall in frustration, and sometimes I didn't sleep. One time I ripped my shirt open, popping all the buttons off, when I was worked up in a private rage and imagining that I was going to fight one of my lieutenants for making us stand an unnecessary inspection.

In my mind at the time, I had no other way to repair these relationships. I was too conflicted and needed to get away from this negativity. I had to defend myself eventually and cut them off by acting as if these people were dead to me—I ignored them as much as I could. I wanted nothing to do with them, as if they didn't matter, just like the cat that I had to strangle and throw away. I was in pain and hurt but finally free from its teeth, from their bullshit.

The black cat dreams told me *loud* but not *clear* that I had to change something, something about me. I didn't know what or how deep I needed to go inside myself to find the answer, though. I thought I was righteous, doing everything right. All I knew was that my leaders had the ability to make me very unhappy. If I didn't want to be unhappy anymore, it was time to go. I needed to leave the Marine Corps and leave the dream that I had lived/loved in the first half of my twenties.

So just as I ran away and into the Marines, I quickly retired my boots and ran away out of the Marines in January of 2000. I knew I had to change the way that I related to people. I couldn't let my anger build up for so long. I needed to communicate more, control my surroundings, and not allow people to disappoint me. I had no idea how to start expressing these desires; I just knew I needed to try.

My Intel shop of ten celebrated my honorable discharge like the end of most Marine enlistments. We had a cookout on one of the quieter sides of the base. All of my Marines were there, including my bosses at the time (officers and senior enlisted), whom I despised. They asked about my future and praised the accomplishments I had accumulated over my six years of service. They even presented me with a plaque that read: *To Sergeant Rooster Pedersen—a real leader of Marines!*

I cried like a baby when I spoke to the group. I was sad, happy, angry, and excited, all at the same time. I was in love with the Marine Corps, with the guys, and with what we had done; and I had strangled many of my experiences. My negativity had hit its peak, thankfully. It was time to go; my time was up. I needed to leave that place. I was disenchanted, conflicted, cocky, and all-knowing—without joy, passion, or love.

Hsssss!

Ahhhh! Why? At least I'm alive. At least I'm free. Why? Ahhhhh!

CHAPTER 10

SO DAMN LUCKY

My heroes are the ones who survived doing it wrong, who made mistakes, but recovered from them.

—Bono

D o you remember "Y2K" (pronounced *why-two-kay*)? If you were born after 1990, you may have to Google it, for chances are likely slim that you do. It's worth noting, though, because Y2K was the introduction that we all had to this century, the new millennium. And to me, looking back, it was also the first real global scare after the Cold War. It also seemed to open a new era of scares. Instead of worrying that thermal nuclear war with the Russians would end the world, Y2K made everyone fear the end of civilization because of global computer failure. I watched the Marine Corps and the entire US government spend billions of dollars from 1998-1999 as they tried to make everything "Y2K compliant." Corporate America and the world followed suit.

You have to remember that every computer in the world was supposed to break at midnight, thereby affecting bank ATMs, utilities, satellites, gas stations, modems, e-mail . . . Even toasters, blenders, and juicers were all supposed to fail. No one knew what mayhem would happen then. Some creative folks speculated that computers would rise up and overthrow the human race with some sort of powerful computer intelligence that we humans wouldn't be able to predict or control. This was the electronic equivalent of El Niño—the nature scare. For several years leading up to midnight, January 1, 2000, terms like *computer crisis, millennium bug, major bug, scare,* and *horror* were used to describe the Y2K time bomb.

I didn't understand it myself. Not being computer savvy at the time, I figured it was just another way for people to worry about another boogeyman. Never one to be caught unprepared, though, I did purchase a gallon of water, three packets of beef jerky, and a pack of bubble bum. Sure, I callously ignored my Marine survival training as the news showed people frantically filling their bathtubs with water and storing rooms full of pork and beans, but I figured that this array of snack food would occupy me during the twelve-hour road trip to St. Louis, Missouri, where I was going to ring in the crashing of the modern world with my big brother, Ben.

When the ball finally dropped in Times Square on New Year's Eve 2000, nothing happened except for a huge celebration. No blackouts occurred, water still ran from our pipes, ATMs still issued my cash, and the New Year's fireworks lit up the winter sky. No major problems were reported either, and the whole world continued with normal life—except for me. I was now freshly out of the Marine Corps and the world I had known for my adult life was over.

I suppose Y2K stands out in my mind because my life seemed to follow the same pattern with intense fear, worry, and overreaction showing up in many crevices of life. Despite my conscious decision to improve my attitude toward people after my black cat nightmares, I still couldn't seem to shake the funk that was deep inside me. I remember trying to be a normal twenty-six-year-old and feeling behind all the other twenty-six-year-olds who didn't go to the Marines. They had graduated college, had regular jobs and were making money, had integrated into society, and had everything—at least, that's what I self-judgingly thought (again/still). I was self-critical of how I dressed, feeling that my fashion sense was way behind the times. I worried that I didn't fit in, that I couldn't relate to the guys or impress the girls.

It's easy to see now how I was subconsciously tapping into my old friend: my limiting pattern of inadequacy. It's painfully true that false worry, blindness to life, and my illusions kept me empty and anxious. Same ole Doug! Apparently, you can run from yourself, or to the Marines, but eventually you run out of breath—and the mirror of life is still there, glaring you in the face when you stop to gasp for air.

Anxiety and deep insecurity (still in me somewhere) were harder to shake than 125 pounds of pure fat. Of course, being a grown man by now, I refused to let people see my vulnerability or know just how small I felt all the time. So of course I responded by overdoing everything (again/still). After stumbling a bit with schools and majors, I finally picked a path and was accepted to the University of Colorado at Boulder. I got my bachelor's in business and finance in just two years and damn near got straight As—how funny is it for a former community college dropout to become *Mr. Dean's List*? The academics were solid in Boulder, but the party scene was stellar, so of course I partied harder than the next guy. Beer wasn't strong enough for me. I favored gin and vodka—sometimes at the same time. I dated for pure lust instead of pure love, joined groups so I didn't feel alone, and I overactivated myself. Like everything else in my bingeing past, in typical Doug fashion, I overdid everything to try to make my inadequacy go away.

Overcompensating in my life's silly situations was my way of doing something about the fears that my obsessions brought out in me. But overcompensating to avoid facing myself (still) just led me back to periods of extreme dissatisfaction and unhappiness. I couldn't even be completely happy when I got my fancy investment banking job after I graduated—or when after a while, I traded in Wall Street to sell millions of dollars' worth of Y2K compliant computers to American companies. No amount of success made a difference to my well-being.

Over the years, I appeared to be living a fine and dandy existence to everyone else in the world. In the end, I had to recognize that I had essentially created these unsatisfying situations. I had to get super honest with myself and acknowledge that I had created my own fear, my own struggle, and my own frustrations. I realized much later that I kept this pattern as a way of connecting with myself. I was chasing significance, trying to feel important, but doing so in the lowest form and most negative ways I could choose to do so. Feeling self-pity was actually meeting my human needs—go figure.

I'm so damn lucky that this veil of illusion eventually started to lift. I even remember exactly when my blindness started to ease: six years after Y2K. It was 2006, and I was thirty-two years old, a former Marine, a college grad, and a road warrior with a big sales territory—ironically selling boatloads for a global computer powerhouse that helped start (and prevent) Y2K. Moreover, I was living in a trendy downtown Chicago loft. I had evolved into a big teenager, even thinking of my company car as a Big Wheel for adults. Still, I was alone and privately unhappy.

For me, 2006 was a pivotal year because that's when my dear grandpa Andy died and when I met my future wife (remember Chapter 1: Like "Nurse" with an "-Iss"?). Something about these two events triggered my third big awakening, which led to another major turning point (the first was losing weight; the second was the cat dream and admitting that I needed to improve my attitude/reactions with people; and now third: seeing life as it really was). Something about experiencing the grief of a death combined with the vulnerability that came from opening my heart to a new, true love stirred the spirit within my soul. It really started me on the conscious path (the quest) of healing, possibility, potential, and might I dare say, wholeness.

I talked about Nurys—the ever-so-smart lovely and beautiful Dominican with eagle eyes—in the opening chapter. She still stirs my heart after six years. Likewise, my grandpa Andy was in my heart. He was an amazing man and someone that I had admired and felt connected to my whole life. Maybe it was because I share his name (my middle name is Andrew), but it was also mainly because he was a very likable and loving family man. Andy was the grandpa who always visited us with a big smile and a huge belly laugh in tow. He also was the grandpa who kept a thick gray beard so he could play Santa Claus in the winter and excite us kids with his deep ho-ho-hos.

He loved his big family, and he truly loved and cared for his wife of sixty years—Grandma Lucy. What a love story! They reared eight children over twenty years; the last one came when Lucy was forty-three years old! Andy was a survivor of the Great Depression, a World War II veteran, a hardworking farmer, a loving father, and a jovial optimist. He was special; I used to believe that they just don't make people like that anymore. I loved him deeper than I ever realized, and although his death was not a surprise, it struck me hard.

Andy spent Y2K in a veteran's hospital in Scottsbluff, Nebraska, a small farm town where he had lived and raised his family (my mom) for many years. He was admitted in 1998 and had spent almost eight years there before he died. I, along with the entire family, stood by and watched Andy deteriorate over that period. He degraded from a man who was larger than life (buttons-popping-off-of-shirt happy) to a patient of the government, sidelined by bouts with skin cancer, pneumonia, and eventually Alzheimer's. The amazing part was that even when he was reduced from using a cane to a walker and then from a walker to a wheelchair, and finally forced to abandon his wheelchair and submit to the permanent confines of a bed, Andy never broke. He never lost his amazing spirit. Even when he lost the ability to speak coherently and carry on with a normal conversation, he seemed to never whine, bitch, or complain—at least not to me.

One day well before he died, my grandpa and a few of the other vets flew the coop and broke out of the hospital. Apparently, they flew their wheelchairs right out the front double doors when the on-duty nurse was distracted. The battery-operated wheelchair must have cranked to full speed as Andy raced across the blacktop parking lot and down the country road that led to the neighboring corn fields. He probably felt liberated as the sun beamed on his wrinkled, bald skin and the country wind filled his aged lungs one more time.

As my mom shared this story with me, I could imagine Andy racing freely down the road like a race car driver. He apparently got a few hundred yards away before the orderlies caught up with him. What joy he must have felt to be free, even if for a moment, from the doctors, the pills, and the sick air inside the hospital room.

Andy was placed on lockdown after this incident—literally! We had a chuckle at the time because Andy was well into his eighties, couldn't even walk, and they made him wear an ankle bracelet as if he were on house arrest. The bracelet activated the doors to shut and lock every time he got near one of them. Not even this little development killed his spirit. If he could talk, I imagine he would say something like, "I would've gotten farther if the chicken hadn't crossed the road right in front of me!" I loved him for this spirit, for this example. What spunk! What heart! There was no quitting in him.

Through updates like this, over time I realized that Andy was much more present in his life than any of us—or at least more than I was. He was living actively within his constraints and limitations, not trying to control them or succumb to them. He was alive; he didn't let the darkest, most depressing circumstances kill his spirit. This made him even more able-bodied, powerful, and wise in my eyes.

My mom and I visited Andy at the VA home several months after his "prison break." I knelt by his wheelchair and razzed him about his stunt. I wanted to laugh with him and let him know that I intended to carry on in my life just as he had. He turned to address me with his eyes, and he surprised me a bit when he tried to talk. Andy could only mumble softly, though. He mumbled to me for maybe five or ten minutes; it seemed like forever as my attention hung on every sound.

My soft-spoken grandma Lucy stood faithfully behind his wheelchair and finally started talking over his mumbles. She smiled like only Lucy Young could and simply said, "Your granddad is proud of you, and he loves you." My skin tingled around my neck, and I felt the emotions begin to build behind my eyes. He was an aging hero who was dying—so genuine, so proud. I felt his love radiating around me.

Eventually I couldn't take it any longer, and I crumbled in place. My legs had fallen asleep from kneeling. I started to cry as I looked in his eyes. I hadn't cried in years, but I broke down like a baby in that moment. Overwhelmed with the circumstances, and somewhat surprised by my own reaction, I stood up and limped out of the room and into the hallway. My mom followed me out, and I latched on to her as I hadn't in decades. We hugged tightly as I cried on her shoulder for what seemed to be another eternity. I was crying for Andy, for Lucy, for my mom, and for myself— deeply saddened by the void his passing would cause in all of our hearts.

For some reason, I really started asking myself the tough questions when Andy finally died. I really started to self-evaluate. Just as I had been sick and tired of being super fat as a kid, I was sick and tired of still feeling super alone and privately unhappy and insecure. So I asked myself, *Why do I feel this way? What have I done to cause this? What can I do differently now in order to change?*

I was in a solemn mood during the holidays that year, the kind of mood that kept me from shaving, talking to many people, and going home to be with family. I suppose you could say that I was soul-searching, scanning, remembering, thinking, and pondering; and although it took time, I finally started to get the answers that I was looking for. And ironically, the answers made me realize that my life, my distorted choices and perceptions, were like a near-death experience I had several years prior, which was way scarier than Y2K.

Several months after I left the Marines, my parents and I drove together from Denver to Omaha to visit my brother. He lived there at the time, and besides having a good family visit, he was going to let me borrow his cherry-red Chrysler Sebring. See, I was back in my parent's house, transitioning into regular-guy civilian life—feeling less than crappy about the silly things I thought I needed but didn't have—and my brother was going to lend me his car until I got into college, got my own place, and found my own car. What a giver my big brother is. Anyway, Ben's Sebring reminded me of my favorite surfboard: sporty and fast but not so good in the snow.

At the end of the visit, we set out on the eight-hour drive back to Denver. Mom and I took the Sebring; I was behind the wheel. My dad took his regular position in the captain's chair of his giant Chevy Suburban. Of course, he was prepared to power through the entire drive without a single pit stop. My mom and I, having done this many times, buckled in and followed him in the *surfboard*. Before long, we entered what was to become a fairly large winter snowstorm. The storm track lasted for about 150 miles and brought lots of fierce wind and wet snow that we were determined to drive through. I was annoyed because I just wanted to get home as quickly as I could.

Everything was normal and very *Nebraska* for the first hour driving into the storm. Despite the gusty snow and the wet roads, traffic moved at a fast pace, and I enjoyed the conversations my mom and I were having. As I traveled down the right lane, I noticed the snow on the road becoming thicker, so I decided to change to the left lane. *No big deal,* I thought. Two big ruts cut down to the pavement from the cars that had already passed. Trust me when I say that no one was thinking *black ice.*

All of a sudden, at eighty-five miles per hour, the car began to fishtail—the rear end shimmied aggressively from side to side. I had never been in this situation, but my instinct told me to steer out of it. I turned the wheel to the right, trying to correct our path by turning to the opposite side of the fishtail. The rear of the car quickly shifted to the left, slipping across the black ice like a huge red windshield wiper. I quickly made another correction, steering the wheel to the left, and the rear end of the car started to slide back and forth along a wider angle. Without time to think, I quickly kept tweaking the wheel, and within seconds, we swung violently to the right and left five or six more times before starting to spin like an eighty-five-mile-per-hour dreidel.

My mom braced herself in the passenger seat. She then lightly reached over and touched my right arm as it clutched the steering wheel. "We're okay. We're okay. Thank you, Lord," she calmly repeated as the car spun us around and around and around.

After several more moments, the car effortlessly spun down the highway and across two lanes of traffic before finally coming to rest in the snow-packed median. My hands and fingertips were locked to the wheel. I could feel the vibrations run through my arms as I sat still, having unsuccessfully controlled the situation. Two semis and a pack of cars roared by our front windshield as we looked at the spot on the road where I had just left my skid marks.

My heart started to beat so fast and so heavy that I thought it was going to pop out of my mouth at some point. The good news was that I could also feel my chest start to constrict like a sphincter, so I knew my heart was going to stay down my throat.

"Holy shit!" I said with a half-fake smirk. "Are you okay, Mama? I'm so sorry. Are you okay? I can't believe we made it out of there without flipping and causing a pileup!"

My mom looked at me with a smirk of her own, and in her own angelic way once again said, "We're okay. We're okay. Thank you, Lord." Her grip eased from my forearm, and we sat in silence looking at each other—taking in the wretched moment we had just experienced. Our eyes were locked as our breathing slowed. We smiled, hugged, and shared a few tears. The profound emotion of what we had just lived through filled the car.

I couldn't help but feel incredibly careless, responsible, blessed, and thankful—all at the same time. I was in a hurry to get back to Denver, and I was more upset that I hadn't taken the proper road precautions with my mom in the car. I saw how I risked her safety when I didn't think much about my own.

Luckily, the car didn't flip, as it surely could have, and by the grace of God, the trailing pack of cars weren't close enough for us to career into as we spun out of control. My mom and I had dodged a tank bullet, and we both knew it. After a few tears and some gentle laughter, I inched the car slowly back onto the highway to catch up with my dad, who was parked several miles down the road, annoyed and wondering where we had gotten off to pee. "Sorry, Dad. I had to stop in the median because I thought I was going to crap my pants."

Sitting there in my airy loft, contemplating my unsatisfying life, I realized that this experience was the same thing I had done with my emotions and my reactions since I was a kid. As with the car, little adjustments back and forth led to big overreactions and bad outcomes. What I should have done in the car is what I should have been doing in life: hold the wheel steady and balanced (ten and two), tap the brakes, and slow my speed down (slow my thoughts and actions down) until I gained control of the car (gained control of myself). I'm so damn lucky that I finally "learned to drive" myself.

I could apply this pattern to many areas of my life. In many instances, I acted cocky, tough, superior, determined, and focused throughout my young and adult life. Deep, deep down, however, I felt extremely inadequate—worried that I would never be loved; worried that I would always be judged by others; worried that I would never be enough. (Like many other people, I'm certain.)

After this beam of light from above, it was easy to see how I had let my rich experiences become empty, shallow, and for nothing. Each of my life's adventures had been like planning a big road trip to the Grand Canyon—being super excited about the adventure, romanced by its reputation for beauty and for being one of the wonders of the world—only to get there and see the glorious canyon as simply just another big hole in the ground, like any other dirty hole in the earth, and feeling disappointed.

I hadn't appreciated my own beauty or my own accomplishments—ever. I never was present with myself, truly comfortable with myself, never sharing my victory over obesity, my accomplishments in the Marine Corps, and my desire to love and live in harmony. I saw the magnificent Grand Canyon as another dirty hole. I saw myself as another dirty hole—and I let my hopes and dreams drop into that hole every time I accomplished a goal and got to my destination. I suffered from my striver mentality and my end-of-the-world syndrome. In the end, this pattern of chasing significance, feeling deep insecurity and overreaction (bingeing to compensate), fit me like a snug Isotoner glove.

My life had the potential to continue swinging wildly from one low-road behavior to the next had I not changed my ways. I'm sure that I would have jumped from one dream job to another, from one city to another, and from one sketchy relationship to another, searching for something I couldn't see or define. I felt freer after receiving this breakthrough when Andy died. Admittedly, being personally accountable in an intense way and becoming an active participant in my own growth was the key to the treasure chest I was looking for a long time. Just like in the Marines, where I learned the principal of participating in your own survival, peace, happiness, and balance were also in my direct control, and I knew that I had to learn how to participate in my own improvement (happiness) if I was ever going to walk this earth with a genuine smile on my face. I'm so damn lucky!

I'm so damn lucky that I finally realized that my brawl with childhood obesity wasn't random. I'm so damn lucky that I finally saw how I easily romanced and blinded myself to life. I was going through life with my *eyes wide shut*! I'm so damn lucky that I lived through Y2K. I'm so damn lucky that the veil over my eyes started to lift in 2006 and I was able to cut my own bullshit. I'm so damn lucky that I finally realized that I was a short-order cook who couldn't stomach his own food.

CHAPTER 11

THAT'S LIFE

Life is one big road with lots of signs. So when you riding through the ruts, don't complicate your mind. Flee from hate, mischief and jealousy. Don't bury your thoughts; put your vision to reality. Wake Up and Live!

—Bob Marley

D o you believe there's a meaning to life? You know, a higher purpose for us people . . . for the world?

Don't get me wrong. My purpose here is not to discuss religion, convince anyone of a certain spiritual belief, or debate or refute anyone's philosophy about life. I do believe, however, that if you're reading this book—for your child or for yourself—and if you've hung in there with my story up to this point—we can likely now agree that life (at least in part) is about learning and teaching lessons, deeply personal lessons.

I'm happy to report that I don't believe for a minute that I've lived a hard life—or that my life has been a complete disaster. In fact, I believe just the opposite. Most of the specific times I've written about in this book outline my deepest feelings and fears about the illusions that I believed at a deep level in my own head, those that held me back from living life happy and free. As I've gained more consciousness, the life lessons have kept rolling into my life like a beautiful tide that gains power with each wave. And for me, life has gotten seriously better and more intense (in a great way) with each tidal set . . . with each of my trips to the *spiritual blackboard*, if you will. It would be a lie to say that these critical life lessons have always come the easy way. Oftentimes they have arrived because of some sort of pain (emotional or physical), struggle, or disappointment. Still, my unquenched thirst to simply understand and do better keeps me curious about how to improve.

It's also important for me to tell you that each life lesson has been followed or includes a benefit (blessing). And there are many more lessons and benefits/blessings that exist than I've talked about or could talk about in this book (outlining every universal lesson/blessing isn't the purpose of *Tuna Breath*—know what I mean?) But trust me when I say that all people should look forward to experiencing problems in their life. Seriously! That's the magic cue—our chance, really—to improve and elevate ourselves. Real learning, real healing, real balance, real fulfillment, and real happiness is standing right in the middle of the storm we think we're in. It's patiently waiting for us like a chauffeur. Let me give some examples.

I'm still disturbed when I remember witnessing a man my age, twenty-nine years old at the time, commit suicide. I was working in San Francisco for an investment bank, walking around trying to act/feel righteous and important. He was doing the same, I later read in the newspaper. It was Christmas Eve when the man wrapped himself from head to toe in a floral bedspread. Directly after this, he leaned forward and fell from the balcony rail on which he was sitting Humpty Dumpty style—from the thirteenth floor of the downtown Marriot. He flew 130 feet down before bouncing six feet up off the concrete directly in front of me and the crowd of people that stood watching him in the minutes before. A firefighter started CPR, but it was clearly a waste of time. It sounds strange to say, but I thank the man for this valuable lesson. I personally hated my life at the time and was very self-centered. This display of self-centeredness helped me realize that selfishness debilitates a person—and it can take many things away from you (including life) while causing pain to those it's pointed at.

My first traumatic breakup was another valuable lesson. It was *Old Yeller* sad and happened a few months after I witnessed the suicide. This is when I felt my heart for the first time. It was so dark and damp, so broken, and so swollen with pain that I didn't sleep more than two hours per night for four months. She was the first serious adult love I had after years of casual hookups with random girls. We met in college, and I had even quit my *important* job in San Francisco to be with her in Denver. We separated just days after I arrived—completely out of the blue and for reasons I thought only the universe could explain. I nearly missed the lesson by trying to escape the pain with as much gin as I could put in my mouth, and with as many girls' phone numbers as I could collect, on a weekly basis. But in time, I realized that my jealousy, domineering personality, and the things I said and did (even only occasionally) as a result of my deep insecurities just weren't attractive to anybody.

I thank God for getting arrested a few months after this breakup. Paying the consequences to the City of Denver for the driving under the influence charges I pled guilty to was a saving grace. Thank God I didn't kill anyone. Getting handcuffed; sitting in a drunk tank talking crazy babble to cops; and then dealing with court, lawyers, community service, fines, alcohol classes, and driving restrictions for almost a year literally jerked my head out of my own ass. I was still working on the selfishness thing, but this episode helped accelerate that process while showing me that there is no escape from pain. There are only ways to deal with pain (positive and negative). We can choose to overcome it or we can choose to succumb to our pain and suffer. Call it "karma" or call it "What goes around comes around." I called it *bullshit* when I blew well over twice the legal limit into the Breathalyzer, but it was simple for even me to understand, after I sobered up, that in this life, in this world, we humans get exactly what we deserve. We reap exactly what we sow, so it behooves us to do things right, be respectful, and to treat ourselves and others extremely well.

A few years later, and after doing a lot more work to balance myself out, is when the real blessings started. Marrying Nurys was the best thing I have ever done. It was, and still is, the absolute best life decision I've ever been fortunate enough to make. My commitment to her has taught me what real love is all about. I now know that real love is played on a level where the participants access and accept that vulnerable space that exists in all of our hearts. It's that space we give from, where we put others first just because we love them, not because we've traded for it or because we expect anything in return. It's the space in our hearts where love is the only reason and the simple reason for doing something/anything for someone else.

Being with Nurys has brought me all the beautiful things in my life. She has brought out the best in me—the most pure sources of growth, contribution, and fulfillment that I have ever known. Without a doubt, Nurys has straightened me out, and God knows where I would have ended up had I continued acting like a douche after our first encounter. We've been together for six, going on seven years now. We own a successful staffing company together and share this life to the fullest. She's my partner in life and in everything I do. No one ever accused us of sitting on the sidelines.

Every moment with Nurys hasn't been full of *pat-a-cake* and *baker's men,* though. We're blessed in many ways, but like many others, we've also been road tested. Our wedding year (2009) was one of them. I spent every penny I made, had ever saved, and could borrow that year. The Great Recession (the world's latest financial scare) threated to swallow our business just as we expanded our operations and opened a new branch office in Washington, DC. We were overextended for sure, and we both put up everything we had to stay afloat despite the risks and uncertainty. It was definitely scary. There were moments where I believed the financial hole we were free-falling into didn't have a bottom. At one point, I believed that it would take us ten years to recover—minimum.

I don't believe we were reckless spenders, but standing on the edge of financial ruin taught me a few things about quitting that high school football never did. I almost quit on our beautiful wedding (not on marrying Nurys). I almost quit on our business venture . . . our future. I almost quit on my dreams of being a successful entrepreneur and helping my wife succeed. But thank God I was guided to hang in there and choose to believe that every problem has a solution . . . even mine. Financial theory teaches that risk is correlated with reward—the higher the risk, the bigger the reward. Thank God I was able to gut it out and see it another way: that every problem, big and small, contains huge amounts of potential for improvement and success. Thank God I learned that instead of running away from problems, we should run to the problem and let our creativity work it out. When we do, we can receive the golden nuggets of success that are waiting for us when we continually elevate our positions.

The huge financial stress of the Great Recession drove me to find new ways to deal with situations that cause eye-twitching pressure. Historically,

I would either exercise or drink my stress away. But meeting a former Chicago Bear (drafted by the Dallas Cowboys in the 1960s) at a stress management workshop in 2010 taught me that there truly are seasons to life—just as there are weather seasons throughout the year. Call it life stages; call it maturing; call it evolution. I called it an "aha moment" when I finally calmed down and let nature take its course in so many areas in my life. I realized that there is an evolution to things; everything we desire has to get planted, then it has to be fertilized, and then it has to grow, just like everything in nature. Our business and personal finances rebounded exponentially in 2011, and we've grown our company 100 percent since those dark days in the winter and spring of 2009. There is a sequence and an order to everything we do, and that long-term perspective I was missing finally got installed . . . *Ohm!*

One of the most valuable lessons I've learned, however, has come from the three miscarriages that Nurys and I have lived through since we've been together. We lost the first one eight weeks in, the second one twelve weeks in, and we lost our third baby at four and a half months into the pregnancy. (More about that in a bit.) Don't get me wrong; miscarrying and losing a baby sucks big time, but I had to find the positive side even in these instances. So by our second loss, I was determined to understand life beyond what a doctor could tell me.

With each pregnancy, Nurys and I experienced the same excitement as most parents-to-be: *We're expecting!* Like many future moms, Nurys subscribed to the baby blogs and kept up to date with our little angel's weekly developments. Many times Nurys would read the developments aloud to me as we sat in bed dreaming about our future family. After hearing the sequence a few times with these pregnancies, and getting through the initial "I'm pregnant" doctor visits with Nurys, it finally dawned on me that we (people) are hearts first. (More on this lesson as well . . . also in a bit.)

Thank God Nurys and I weren't permanently discouraged by our losses. Like many other couples that have miscarried, we finally were blessed with a healthy baby. Fatherhood has taught me many lessons—and more are expected—but up to now I can say that the birth of our son, Andrew Silvano, in 2011 helped me understand and really feel unconditional love. Contributing to the health, well-being, and growth of an innocent beautiful young child is a source of fulfillment that I didn't realize I was depriving myself of. It's so natural. He's fourteen months old at the time of this writing. I'm so fortunate to have been able to be home with him a great deal during his first year on the planet. Our relationship is awesome, and he's the coolest dude I know. I love hanging out, playing, reading, and teaching him where his hair, nose, teeth, and ears are. But I'm most proud that my little man also knows where his heart is—true story.

Can you believe that I actually told people for thirty-four years that I didn't think I would ever have kids? I even told Nurys that I was sterile when we first started dating. The Navy doc that did my final physical said there would be a chance of that, and I found it easy to avoid family responsibility that way. What a *chooch* move, but I didn't even know what I was missing until I met my son, Andrew. The light literally changed in the delivery room the minute he popped out—for Nurys and me anyway.

Likewise, the birth and death of my second son, Allen William, in 2012 once again reaffirmed the lesson of unconditional love. Allen was a beautiful baby, and we lost him in the fourth month of pregnancy. Losing him the way we did was the hardest thing I've ever faced. The grief in my heart went way deeper than anything I've ever experienced. It's like having your heart removed with a baseball bat. But growing, evolving, and elevating my spirit all this time allowed me to demonstrate my faith in that difficult moment. Losing Allen affirms my belief that there really is a divine plan that leads us. Allen was part of our plan, part of our evolution, and part of what heals our past and draws our love closer together today and every day since. *You are loved, Allen William Pedersen!*

So what was my point/lesson with the "we are hearts first" business? Well, it sounds weird to say (and I do this on purpose), but when I say that we are hearts first, I literally mean that before we human beings develop fingers, toes, eyes, or any major organs, we get our hearts and our heartbeats first! The heart is the first major organ to "appear" and is formed in week six of the pregnancy. Before that, we're merely biological material—cells that contain genetic coding and such. But in week six, the heartbeat is magically present, *feeling*, and pumping away twice as fast as the carrying mother's.

"What about the brain?" you ask. Well, did you know that while the heart is doing its thing in week six, the brain is nowhere to be found? In fact, the brain isn't fully formed until week twelve—and most importantly, it doesn't receive the full set of neurons (those things needed for memory and so forth) until we are six months old (yes, that's out of the womb—feel free to check it all out on www.babycenter.com or www.baby2see.com). So while the brain is taking its time trying to figure out how it's going to work, the heart is doing its thing. We are truly and literally hearts first!

This is one reason these miscarriages were so valuable to me. Among other things, tracking the pregnancies and analyzing our troubling situation over and over again helped me to see and validate that our hearts are the true sources of intelligence. Not our brains. Many of us follow our logical brains (as I did for so long), but it's really the feelings in our hearts that run the show. The brain isn't even second in the development line and doesn't even get its first memory until it's out of the womb for six months. But the heart has been beating, feeling, and knowing strongly for at least fifteen months at that point.

The heart is first, and the heart *always* knows what's best for us—so it pays to follow it. And ultimately, what does the heart represent? It represents love, and that's who we are. We're hearts (love) first and at our cores. Everything else—fear, struggle, insecurity—is simply learned information in the brain and is not who we are. Those bits of information act as our illusions, and we can grow out of (literally shake out of) the illusions if we're open and willing to get back to our source—back to what we naturally know . . . back to our hearts.

Could this be the true meaning or purpose to life? Well, others can debate that. I know, however, that following my heart is one of my life's goals. By reading my story, I hope you can see how I do this—by opening myself to learning, even the hard way. I call this process "LIFE" (used as an acronym). LIFE presented this way simply means this: Look Inward First Every time for answers to any life problem or scenario.

LIFE has taught me about physical and emotional balance. LIFE reveals the true intentions of my heart. When I LIFE, I learn about my illusions and see how I've distorted the truth; I learn about choices and consequences. LIFE has taught me my needs, my source, my path, my drive, and the drive of others. The beautiful part is that life has literally taught me to LIFE—like when I've been unsatisfied, experienced problems, felt inadequate, been destructive, harmed myself, criticized others, suffered, or when I've just been plain unhappy. You know . . . everything I've already admitted. *Looking inward first every time* I have a *problem* always brings me back to peace, understanding, and happiness—always!

LIFE provided me with the process and answers that I was seeking for so long, and LIFE has helped me break free and break out of my most unsatisfying or unjust life situations. Now I'm confident that life becomes much easier once we finally take personal accountability for our actions; ask ourselves the tough questions; humble ourselves enough to learn basic lessons; attach powerful, positive meaning to things; and simply agree to LIFE and follow our hearts. At the end of the day, the end of this story, I now know on a visceral level never to be scared, fearful, or worried anymore. Why? Because when I look below my chin, I remember that I'm a heart first—and I love more freely, more often.

Now that's one more step to knowing.

Now that's *life!*

PICTURE DIARY

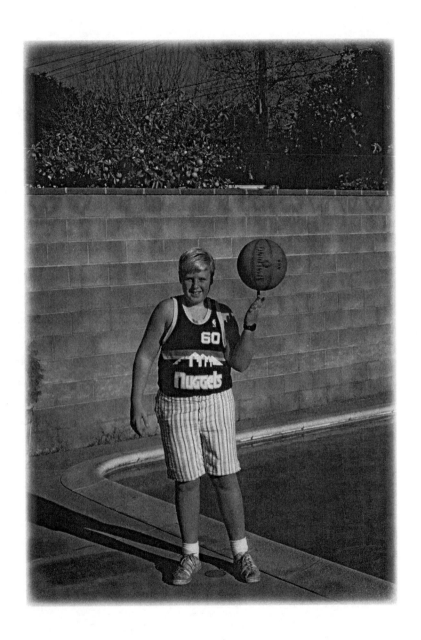

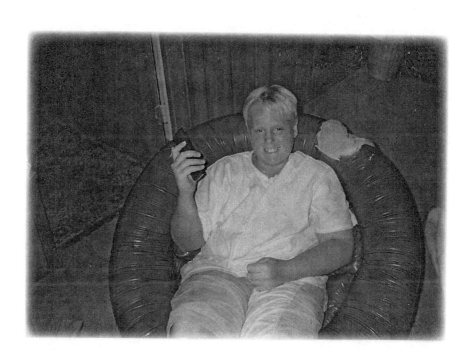

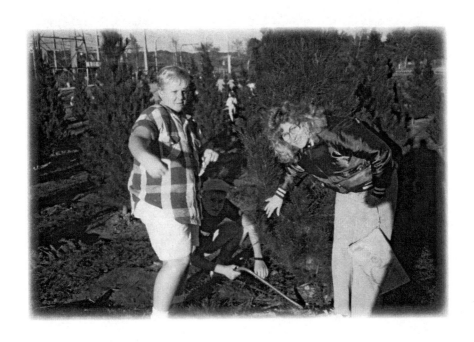

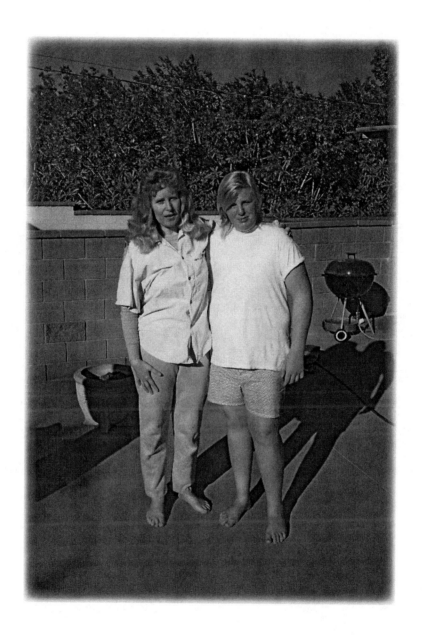

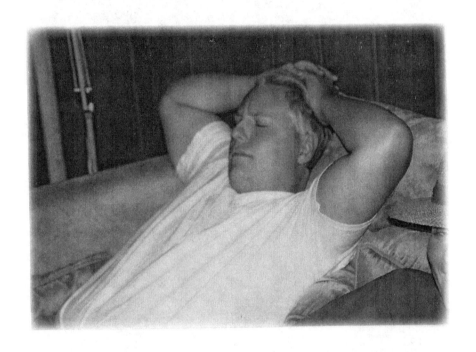

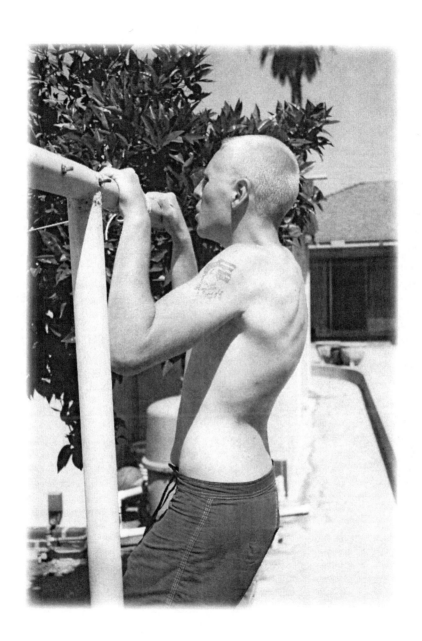

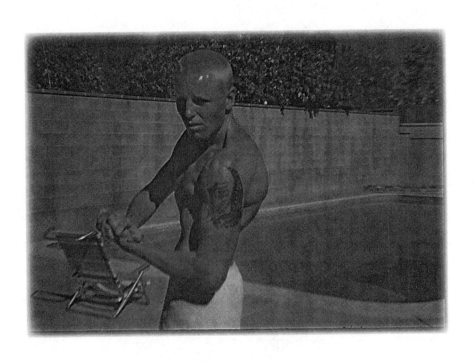

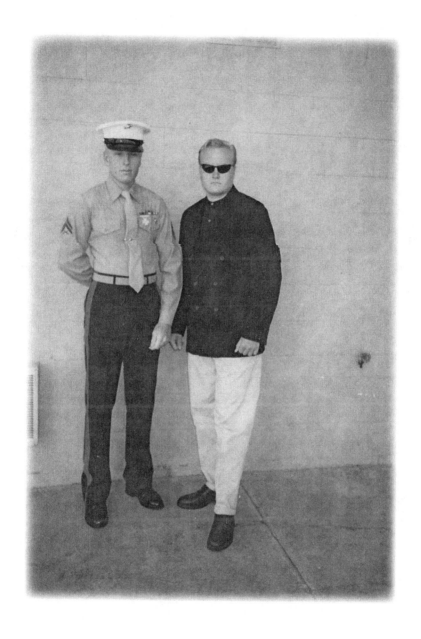

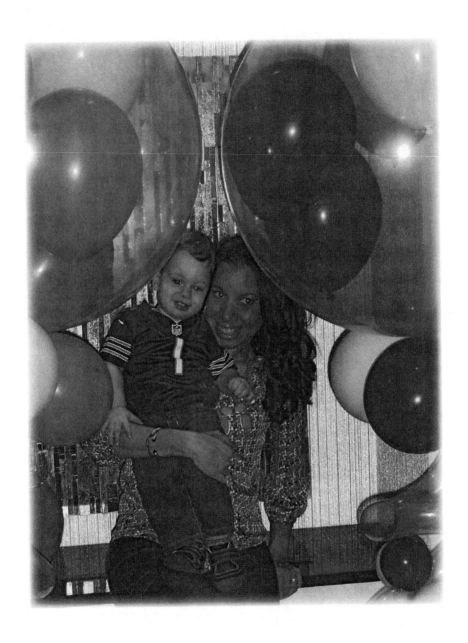

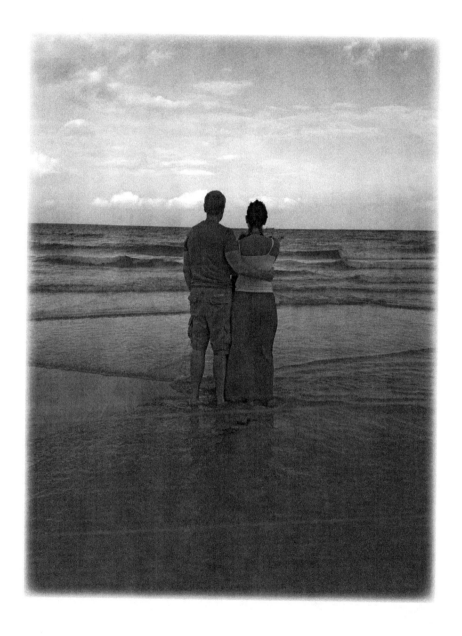

ABOUT THE AUTHOR

Doug Pedersen is a strategic interventionist and founder of PLAYGROUND:GLOBAL, a research and education company. His own history with childhood obesity and study of human nature fuels his writing, speech topics, and teachings, which are designed to help people understand and meet their human needs in balanced, effective, and healthy ways. In his latest project, Doug is helping mothers understand, communicate, and heal their seriously overweight children. Doug currently lives with his wife and son in the Washington, DC area. Visit him at www.dougapedersen.com.

CPSIA information can be obtained at www.ICGtesting.com
Printed in the USA
BVOW03s0135250713

326794BV00003B/11/P